BAD BACK

BAD BACK
Coping for Life

Lucy M. Dobkins

Forewords by
Manuel Lujan, Jr.
William Krieger
Thomas K. Sims

Illustrations by
Robert S. Partch

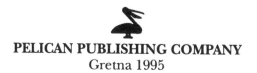

PELICAN PUBLISHING COMPANY
Gretna 1995

Library of Congress Cataloging-in-Publication Data

Dobkins, Lucy M.
    Bad back : coping for life / by Lucy M. Dobkins ; forewords by
Manuel Lujan, Jr., William Krieger, Thomas K. Sims ; illustrations
by Robert S. Partch.
      p.   cm.
    Includes bibliographical references and index.
    ISBN 1-56554-062-X
    1. Dobkins, Lucy M.—Health.   2. Spinal canal—Stenosis—
Patients—United States—Biography.   3. Backache—Patients—
United States—Biography.   I. Title.
    RD771.S74D63   1995
    362.1'97564'092—dc20
    [B]   94-41901
                                                   CIP

*The conversations in this book were not recorded and printed verbatim.
The intent of the author, however, was to present their essence here.*

Manufactured in the United States of America
Published by Pelican Publishing Company, Inc.
1101 Monroe Street, Gretna, Louisiana 70053

To Stanford Hall
for giving me so many reasons
to get well, and helping me do it

CONTENTS

Foreword...9

Preface 13

Acknowledgments 15

Chapter 1   Josi, Help Me!......................................21

Chapter 2   A Normal Recovery: Awful 35

Chapter 3   You May Never Walk Again 41

Chapter 4   Ted's Career Is Ruined, Poor Guy...................49

Chapter 5   And Now What? 55

Chapter 6   A New Beginning 63

Chapter 7   Bad Back: Coping for Life 73

Chapter 8   Life, How Can You Be So Perverse? 87

Chapter 9   Prayers by Fiber-Optic Cable 97

Chapter 10   Please, God, Let It Be in Time 105

Chapter 11   Maybe a Psychologist Can Help 111

Chapter 12   One Down and One to Go 117

Chapter 13   Anterior Spinal Fusion...........................129

Chapter 14   Turning the Corner 141

Chapter 15   Home for Easter...................................147

Chapter 16   You'll Think You're
             Superwoman Again 157

Chapter 17   Santa Fe 167

Chapter 18   Two Steps Forward and
             One Step Back 175

Chapter 19   I Don't Know What Else We Can Do.............185

Chapter 20   Dear Abby......................................189

Chapter 21   Coping Emotionally 193

Chapter 22	Coping Physically	199
Chapter 23	Coping Socially	207
Chapter 24	Coping Financially	209
Chapter 25	Sure, You Can Travel Though Handicapped!	211
Chapter 26	Image Becomes Reality	217
	Suggested Reading	221
	Suggested Listening for Relaxation	225
	Suggested Videos for Relaxation	229
	Index	231

FOREWORD

Lucy Dobkins' story is one of strength. She captures in graphic terms the perseverance of the human spirit.

There are few people who have not experienced back pain at one time or another. The author takes us step by step through her illness. By understanding what she endured, we can better understand ourselves.

Most touching for me is the section where she has to give up her business for her health. It is a decision not easily made, but one that ultimately gives her the proper time to recover. Having had to adjust my life-style for health, I had great empathy for her condition.

This book is both interesting and informative. I cheered when she finally felt strong enough to go back to work, and I felt her pain when a nurse asked her, "You want to walk, don't you?"

Bad Back: Coping for Life will give you the skills necessary to deal with back pain. Lucy's recovery can benefit us all.

THE HONORABLE MANUEL LUJAN, JR.
Former United States Secretary of the Interior;
Former United States Congressman

As a mental health counselor and occupational disability evaluator, I deal on a daily basis with people in pain—people whose lives are devastated by debilitating illness, the aftermath of radical surgery, and the psychological trauma of dealing with the new reality of their lives. Lucy Dobkins' story is not unique; Lucy Dobkins is.

This is a book that needed to be written—not for those who suffer debilitating pain but for those who don't. The real story in this book is not about the pain and suffering of one individual; it is about friendship and caring and loving. It is about the responsibility we, as human beings, have to each other.

My teacher, Dr. George Keppers, one of the early leaders of the counseling profession, kept a sign on his desk that read: *Neither to condemn nor to condone, but to understand.* Lucy's willingness to share her pain and suffering, her lost careers and broken dreams, her psychological depression and loss of faith, is the vehicle by which we are led to understand.

To understand is to enhance our ability to care—to fulfill our responsibility to be a friend. The presence of so many caring, giving friends in Lucy's life is a tribute to Lucy's uniqueness.

WILLIAM KRIEGER, ED.D.
Past Chairman of the National Academy of
    Certified Clinical Mental Health Counselors;
Past President of the American Mental Health
    Counselors Association

God provides food for all the birds of the air,
But he doesn't throw it into their nests for them.

Pain, be it physical or emotional, presents the greatest challenge to the human being. We become our own worst enemies while in pain and experience the gamut of unpleasant human emotions, from depression to despair; from apathy to anger.

Medicine has risen to this challenge with a remarkable array of scientific and technological weapons with which to fight pain. Psychology has increasingly added to the arsenal, too, with increasing knowledge about the mental mechanisms of pain control. The more we advance, though, the more we are forced to return to a recognition and an acceptance of our basic human experience. The effectiveness of our advanced weapons against pain clearly rests upon our basic humanness to make them work.

As a child, I was taught about evil, and a bad back most certainly is evil. I was also taught about good and the basic human truth that virtue is the greatest weapon against evil. This volume is about the three most basic virtues of faith, hope, and love and their power in combating pain.

In the pages of this book, as one walks with Lucy Dobkins in her battle with pain, one sees the emergence of these virtues as powerful weapons indeed. She grows from a woman with a tremendous and healthy faith in herself to a more complete person with faith in her God and in her fellow human beings.

Hope is a constant in this journey, with all the ups and downs and triumphs and defeats that are the hallmarks of hope in all of us. The gift of hope given to her by others and the gift of hope that she returns to them is powerful in its message.

It is the love, however, the greatest virtue of all, that shines most brightly in the book. The love of humans for each other is what makes the more sophisticated weapons work. In the hands of a skilled surgeon, a skilled housekeeper, or simply a skilled friend, love carries the battle forward.

This is a volume for all of us to read. For the person who suffers pain it provides a great many possibilities for victory. For the person who works to heal pain, it provides a strong reminder to always combine one's knowledge with one's humanity. For everyone it serves as a reminder that we are all in this together.

THOMAS K. SIMS, PH.D.
Clinical Psychologist, Behavior Therapy Associates;
Clinical Faculty Member, Department of Psychology, University of New Mexico

PREFACE

Bad Back: Coping for Life is the true story told as it happened to a woman who was successful in her profession, but suddenly had to learn all about spinal problems, terminology, and treatments, and under critical circumstances had to have multiple back operations in a short period of time. As the reader, you will learn while I learn how a myelogram, an MRI exam, a bone scan, and a CT scan are given and how they make you feel. You'll watch me experience the torment of sympathetic dystrophy, compressed nerves, and degenerated discs. My orthopedic surgeon and neurosurgeons will explain to me how they do nerve root decompressions and spinal fusions. I will take you with me into Intensive Care, and you'll feel all the misery I feel.

During my fight to regain my health, I have to give up my profession, and then, after I recuperate and start a new business, I lose that, also to a bad back. I lose my active life-style, my faith in God, and my hope in the future. My medical costs rise to about $500,000, with a loss of probably a million dollars in future earnings.

In this story I learn techniques for coping with chronic, long-term pain, and strategies for adjusting to overwhelming losses. I learn new and better ways of taking care of myself, practicing the suggestions my psychologist makes for relaxing, pacing myself, and protecting my body from physical stresses as he assists in rehabilitating me. I rise from my personal disaster and build a new and happy life and a renewed faith in God.

During these experiences, I learn more about love and loyalty than I have ever known.

On any given day, 6.5 million American men and women are in bed with lower-back pain. *Bad Back: Coping for Life* is written with the hope that the reader will be drawn into it and will gain an increased knowledge about the resiliency of the human spirit, information about back problems and their impact on life, ways to adjust to changes in life-style, and strategies for coping with pain.

It can be difficult to learn a new and different way of life constructed to accommodate physical limitations, but this book can serve as a guide, a guide to coping for life.

ACKNOWLEDGMENTS

The friends, business associates, and members of my family who began talking to me about what I should do with my life once I got out of the hospital didn't wait till I could walk, prepare my own meals, or stop grieving over the store I used to have. Not one of them saw the mountains of obstacles that I saw piled in my way to starting a new life now that the old one wouldn't work.

My sister, long in the medical field, asked, out of the blue, "When are you going to start your book?"

"What book?"

"The book about backs, so other people won't have to learn it all the hard way. They ought to have a chance to know all the things you learned about back problems and how they affect a person's business and personal life."

So, timidly and quietly (who do I think I am to write a book?), I reviewed the personal daily journals of the medical experiences I'd had with my back, studied bundles of notes, conferred with medical specialists to confirm the accuracy of the medical information, consulted medical texts, interviewed other back patients, wrote an outline and developed the story *Bad Back: Coping for Life*.

I want to express my affection and appreciation to all the medical people, friends, and members of my family who helped me get well, those who encouraged me to write this book, and the extraordinary staff at Pelican Publishing Company.

Among them are:

Helen Zitoli, my sister, for convincing me that other people need to know what I have learned about back problems and the impact they can have, and for her constant love.

Dr. David and Jim Zartman, my brothers, and Micki and Margaret, my sisters-in-law, for their steady support.

Terry and Rusty Dobkins, my sons, and Nancy Ney and Judy, my daughters-in-law, for their never-ending love and encouragement during the time that I felt terrible and even now that I am so much better.

Mary Kitchel Zartman, my mother, for her love and indomitable spirit. She is an inspiration to all of us, regardless of her recent death.

Elmer C. Sproul, our family friend, for believing that I can successfully do anything that I set out to do, and for always encouraging me.

My silent partner in Lucy's Pillowtalk for giving me the chance of a lifetime to rebuild my financial future.

Stanford Hall (not his real name) for being the finest, most patient and loving man I've ever known.

Wess Barrow, my treasured friend for more than thirty years, for helping me in so many ways to get through a bad time.

Dee Foster, always my friend and confidante, but especially so when I was in the depths of despair.

Beatrice and Barnett Bittner, for always being my anchors in a stormy sea; and Barnett, translator and writer, for conscientiously and meticulously editing the first draft of this manuscript.

The ministers and members of the First United Methodist Church for their prayers during all the operations, especially when I gave up.

Pat Kroken, successful advertising executive, for convincing me that this book was one that needed to be written and that I was the one to do it.

Eileen Stanton, writer, for evaluating the first manuscript and reviewing it with me line by line. She fueled me with the enthusiasm and confidence to begin the rewrite.

Mary Lynn, writer, for critiquing the first manuscript and making invaluable suggestions.

Denise Bradley, writer, for knowing the answers to my questions about writing this type of book.

The Honorable Manuel Lujan, Jr., United States Congressman,

who had to change his life-style, too, because of a health condition, for understanding what it was like for me, and for writing the foreword for this book; his eternally optimistic wife, Jean, and their son, Jeff, who was my office student aide when I was a counselor.

Dr. William Krieger, Vice-Chairman of the National Academy of Certified Clinical Mental Health Counselors, for his leadership in counselors' organizations, and for writing the foreword.

Dr. Thomas K. Sims, Clinical Psychologist, for being the consulting psychologist for some of my most difficult cases, and for his gracious foreword.

Dr. Reid Hester, my psychologist, who had complete confidence in my future even if I didn't.

Robert S. Partch for his incomparable medical illustrations.

Dr. Milburn Calhoun, owner and president of Pelican Publishing Company; Nina Kooij, editor, wise beyond her years; Jan Fehrman, Western marketing director, for discovering me; and the entire remarkable staff.

Drs. Sidney Schultz and Lloyd Hurley, my orthopedic surgeons, and their staff, for their years of kind and conscientious care.

And especially—

Dr. Sidney Schultz for reviewing the medical passages in this manuscript, and for always doing everything within his power to make me well. It's nice that he knows all about my bones and likes me anyway.

Dr. Steven N. Copp at Scripps Clinic in La Jolla, California, for keeping my spine functioning after Dr. Schultz retired.

BAD BACK

Chapter 1

JOSI, HELP ME!

"Josi, help me!" I cried as I stumbled, pale and shaking, into the nurse's office and sank into the chair she quickly pulled forward. With alarm on her face she demanded, "What happened? What's wrong?"

Josi Hilgers, the tall, blond, no-nonsense nurse at the junior high school where I was a guidance counselor, and I had made an early start on the day and it was not yet eight o'clock on this winter morning. I had gone to my office at seven o'clock to prepare for a heavy schedule of conferences and also to deliver to a classroom a box of test materials a teacher requested. I wanted to do that while the halls were empty and quiet. I went into the file room, pulled from the drawers the test manuals, booklets, and answer sheets needed, and packed them in a box. I picked up the box and carried it out of the counseling suite into the hall to the Language Arts Department.

Suddenly, with no warning, something happened in my back that stunned me! Pain so intense and sharp that I couldn't get my breath engulfed me. I saw that it wasn't going to be possible to reach the classroom and sit down there, but the nurse's office was nearby so I headed for that. I dropped the box of booklets, leaned against the wall, and painfully edged my way to the nurse.

Between gasps of breath I told Josi what had happened and moaned, "I don't know what's wrong."

Knowledgeable about back injuries, Josi quickly evaluated me and determined that this was a case for outside emergency care. She informed the principal what had happened, called an ambulance, notified St. Joseph Hospital that she was bringing me to the emergency room by ambulance, and phoned the orthopedic surgeon who had taken care of me at a previous time to let him know I was going to St. Joseph and why. He said he'd meet us there.

The ambulance, paramedics, and police arrived at the nurse's office. "You've got a problem here?"

Josi brought them to me, explained the circumstances, and said, "We need to take her to the emergency room at St. Joseph Hospital. I don't know what the problem with her back is, so I don't want to do anything that aggravates it. Can you transport her without moving her out of the position she's in now? It's very painful for her to move at all, and it might cause more damage if she does move."

"First, we'll have to take her vital signs," the paramedics said. My pulse and blood pressure were zooming, they soon found out, and I was shaking violently and uncontrollably.

The paramedics adjusted their gurney to make it lower and easier to transfer me to, and raised the head of it to be almost exactly the same angle as the way I was sitting.

The chief paramedic said, "We think we can keep her almost exactly the same if we'll just lift her gently from the chair to the gurney at this height."

With infinite care they lifted me onto the gurney, strapped me securely, covered me with a warm blanket, and rolled me out of the building to the ambulance.

By that time the school was filled with students on their way past the nurse's office to their classes. They had seen the emergency vehicles on the driveway in front of the school and were excited and curious about what was going on. Now, seeing their counselor wrapped and strapped to a gurney and being taken away, their faces showed alarm and concern. I didn't know which was worse: the excruciating pain in my back, or the commotion and upset this was causing our students.

It was the morning rush hour on the freeways in Albuquerque, my town of about a half a million people. Nevertheless, the drive to the hospital was speedy and brief. Josi rode beside me in the ambulance, while the paramedics continually monitored my pulse and blood pressure.

In the emergency room Josi waited with me for Dr. Sidney Schultz to arrive from surgery. When he got there he asked both of us questions, made an examination, and said he wanted me admitted to the hospital. "We're going to need a bone scan, a CT scan, spinal X rays, chest X rays, and blood tests. We'll get started on them right now. After you do the tests, you can get settled in your room and rest. When the results are ready, I'll go over them with the radiologist and let you know what we find."

The nurses in the emergency room transferred me to another gurney, and an escort wheeled me to the Radiology Department. The room we entered was filled with computers, monitor screens, and heavy, specialized X-ray tables. The X-ray technician greeted me cheerily, then said, "The first X ray we're going to do is the CT scan. You don't need to wear a hospital gown for this test, so just stay in the clothes you're wearing."

"A CT scan, or computerized tomogram," he began in explanation, "is a series of X-ray pictures that look at cross sections of different levels of the spine, like when you slice a bologna. You can look at slices that show the vertebrae, discs, areas where the nerves come out of the spinal column, and the surrounding muscles and bowels. The X rays allow the radiologist to look for pathology in the spine. You won't have to do a thing, and you won't feel anything. We just want you to lie perfectly still throughout the time the X rays are being made."

It was necessary for me to lie flat on my back for what seemed like thirty or forty minutes, and the pain was almost paralyzing when I had to keep my back and legs flat against the hard table.

When the CT scan was completed, the technician said, "Now I need to take some chest X rays and X rays of your lower back, so you'll need to change into a hospital gown. I'll get one of the nurses to help you. Don't move any more than you have to."

He helped me off the X-ray table, every move so painful that I thought I'd faint. The nurse helped me change clothes, stayed with me while the X rays were made, and then called an escort to take me to another department for blood tests.

"After they draw your blood, they'll bring you back to us. We're going to draw a syringe of spinal fluid out of your spinal cord so that Dr. Schultz can rule out any possibility of disease in your spine. We're also going to give you an injection of radioactive material in preparation for a bone scan. We'll tell you more about it when you get back."

It took only a few moments for a technician to draw the blood sample, and the escort returned me to Radiology.

The technician was waiting. "We're going to draw the syringe of spinal fluid now, so I want you to lie down on your tummy on this table. You'll feel a little stick from the needle, and then a moment later I'll insert a syringe between two vertebrae and draw the fluid. It won't hurt you much. Just be sure and lie still while I do it."

He injected the needle, drew the spinal fluid, and withdrew the needle quickly and smoothly.

"This next study is a bone scan," he said now. "I'm going to give you an injection of radioactive material and then send you to your room for three hours. At the end of the three hours, you'll be brought back to Radiology for more X rays. This time we'll photograph the radioactive fluid as it travels throughout the passages in your body, and you can watch it on the monitors you see here. That'll give us information about any 'hot spots,' diseased areas, in your bones."

Exhausted and teary, I received the injection and was ready for the escort to take me upstairs to the Orthopedic Floor and check me into a room.

Solicitously, careful to keep from hurting me more, the orthopedic nurses settled me into the room to rest and wait.

Not knowing what was wrong or whether or not it was serious, and not having any idea what would come next, I didn't phone my friends to tell them where I was, and since the only family I had living in town was my elderly mother, I didn't let her know either. There was no use in raising needless anxieties, I thought. There would be time enough to talk with them after Dr. Schultz gave me more information.

Time dragged. I fretted about the appointments being canceled at my office. I reconstructed, moment by moment, the morning of lifting and carrying the box of test materials and tried to identify anything that could have caused the problem. I worried. I hurt—a lot!

After three hours, an escort came to get me and wheeled me to Radiology for the bone scan. It was fascinating to watch on the screens the dark radioactive fluid circulate throughout my body. It didn't take long for the X rays to be completed, and it didn't hurt except for having to move from gurney to table and back, and having to lie flat again.

The bone scan completed, the escort returned me to my room to wait for the radiologist and Dr. Schultz to read the studies, discuss them, and determine what needed to be done.

It was early evening when Dr. Schultz, slender, impeccably dressed, and sporting a neatly trimmed beard and mustache, came to my room to talk about the test results. "The radiologist and I have studied all of your X rays and the spinal fluid," he began. "The good news is that there isn't any evidence of disease in your spine. The bad news is that the studies show that you do have spinal stenosis. You don't have any disc, which is a cushion, between your lumbar vertebrae No. 4 and 5. Those vertebrae, 'joints,' as we call them, are pounding against each other and the nerves. Every time you move, you crush those nerves."

Dr. Schultz was easy to talk to, I'd learned in the past, and he always answered fully any questions I asked him.

"What exactly is spinal stenosis?" I asked.

"Spinal stenosis is a narrowing of the size of the spinal canal and the size of the holes between vertebrae through which nerves emerge from the spinal canal. It can be caused by arthritic bony overgrowth, thickening of ligaments, mal-alignment of vertebrae, or a combination of them."

"What do we do about it?" I asked apprehensively.

"The appropriate treatment is to do a spinal fusion. Do you remember the spinal fusion we did in your neck after you got hit at an intersection? This will be much the same. We'll make a *J*-shaped incision down your lower back at the lumbar 4-5 level and move all the muscles aside so that we can see your spine and work on it. We'll remove any fragments of broken disc and other debris that might be there so that the space between the joints is clean. Then, we'll roughen up the vertebrae and drill

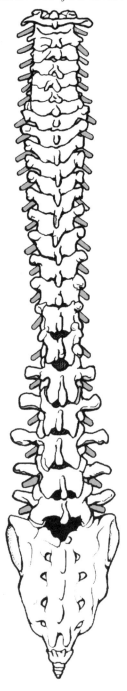

A posterior view of the human spine.

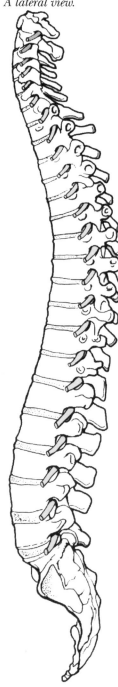

A lateral view.

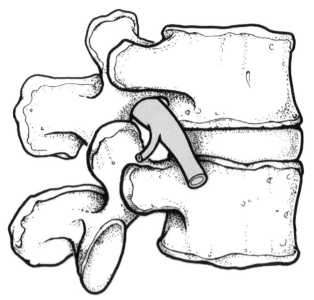

Properly spaced lumbar vertebrae: normal disc and nerve.

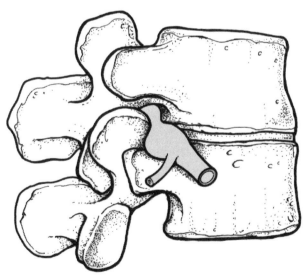

Degenerated, narrowed disc trapping the nerve (spinal stenosis).

Cross section of vertebra and spinal cord.

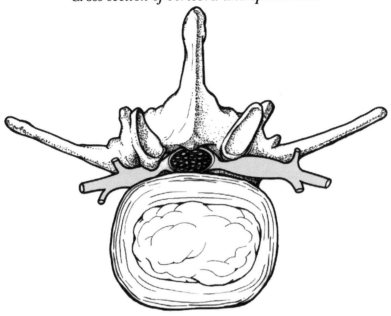

Nerve entrapped (spinal stenosis).

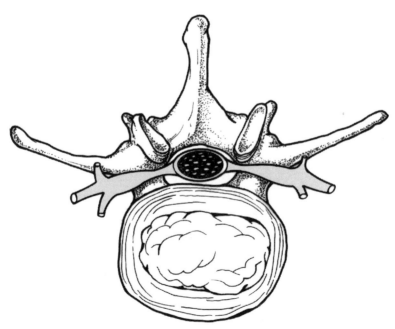

Normal vertebra, spinal canal, and nerve.

a one-inch hole between them. Next, we'll use a mallet and chisel to shave splinters of bone off your hipbone—your ilium. We'll layer those splinters around the holes we've made in your spine and pack them like a beaver builds a dam to form one strong solid mass, a fusion of two vertebrae. They'll then become one solid bone with no movement in them.

"I want to suggest that we implant an electronic device called an Orthofuse. It's like a small battery about the size of your little finger, and it has four electrical wires leading from it. The device is implanted in your back below the lowest rib, and the four wires are placed in the areas which need most to be healed. The theory is that diseased or damaged tissue does not accept the passage of fluids and nutrients between the cells as well as healthy tissue does, and that electrical currents encourage and stimulate bone growth by increasing the flow of fluids. The lifetime of the battery is about six months, and it will be removed in outpatient surgery at that time. If you do want to try it, you'll need to sign a permission form."

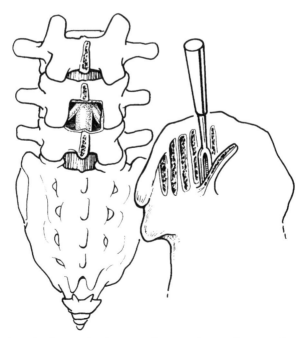

In surgery for spinal stenosis, the spaces between the vertebrae are cleaned and enlarged, and splinters of bone are harvested from the ilium.

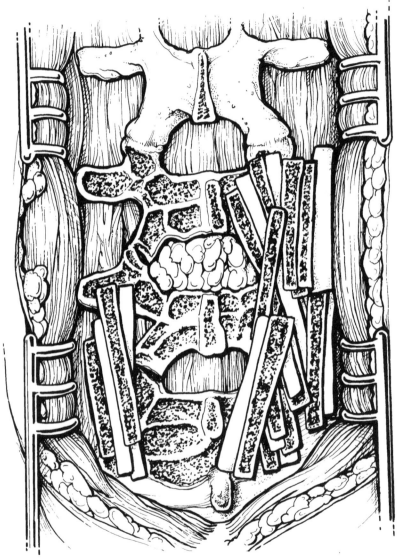

The spine is packed with bone splinters to form a solid fusion.

"If we do this operation," I asked, "how long will I be in the hospital? How long will I be away from work?" My mind panicked with thoughts of the work that would pile up, the students who wouldn't be taken care of, and the extra work load my colleagues would have to absorb on top of their already heavy duties.

"You can expect to be in the hospital about ten days. You can drive a car in six weeks. In three to four months, depending on how fast you heal, you can go back to work part time, but you won't be allowed to do any lifting, reaching above your shoulders, bending down, or sitting or standing for any length of time," Dr. Schultz explained.

"How can I do that?" I demanded to know. "My school is in a good neighborhood, but we have on the fringes of the district three poverty pockets that have the highest rate of major crime in the city. Many of the children I work with live surrounded by fights, theft, drugs, alcohol, neglect, and abuse. For example, one student, Angie, hasn't gone home for two nights because she saw her mother's boyfriend rob and kill the barber down the street, and he knows she saw him do it. Angie's afraid he'll kill her, too, before the police catch him. Another student, Tim, will be back from Texas tomorrow. He was sent there to testify about a murder he witnessed. Jim, a twelve-year-old, is having a terrible time in school since his father shot his brains out in front of him during the Christmas holiday. There are three child abuse cases I'm working on, and the nurse and I have documented all the beatings and burnings. The cases are almost ready to take to court, but they can't be rushed to court before they'll stand up before a judge and jury, or we'll cause more harm than good. If I'm not at school to be available to those children, the chances are that the cases will be dropped. How can I possibly be gone at this time?"

"I can't make your decisions for you, but how good a job are you going to do for those kids the way you're feeling now?" Dr. Schultz asked, putting it into perspective.

Filled with anxieties, I asked, "If we do a spinal fusion, what condition will my back be in after it's over? Will it be ruined forever like others I've heard about?"

"How well did your neck do after the cervical spinal fusion?" Dr. Schultz asked.

"It did perfectly. I've never had another problem."

Dr. Schultz responded confidently, "I think you can antici-pate the same good results with your lower back. Neither the radiologist nor I see anything in the studies to indicate any other problems."

Still resisting, I asked, "What alternatives are there? How about a chiropractor? Acupuncture? Traction? Or physical ther-apy and swimming? How about heat and ice packs? A corset or a cast? Those injections of papaya extract I've heard about? Muscle relaxants? Or the needle that can siphon out crumbs of broken discs and clean up the spine?"

Patiently, kindly, yet firmly, the doctor explained. "There really aren't any good alternatives for this condition. You don't have any cushion between the lumbar vertebrae 4 and 5, so the nerves will continue to be irritated every time you move. The way to stop the irritation is to immobilize the vertebrae."

Dr. Schultz had gained my trust and respect six years earlier when he had done the cervical fusion, and through the years since then I had returned to him from time to time with little problems like stress fractures in my feet, and once a broken toe, but nothing serious. My hesitations now were simply to be sure that a spinal fusion was the best answer, and also the dread of disrupting my life and work as drastically as a spinal fusion can do, not to mention the pain that is a part of back operations.

I came to a decision. "Yes, I'll have the fusion based on the fact that I can't work with my back the way it is now, but I will be able to work after it's repaired."

"I'll go study the operating schedule and find out when we can do the surgery," said Dr. Schultz, standing up to leave. "I'll be back later this evening to let you know."

I lay in the darkening room, hurting, lonely, and apprehen-sive. There were some good things going for me, I realized. There had been a long period of time in which I hadn't been sick or absent from work, so I'd accrued enough sick leave to last a year or more and that would keep my job and income secure. My medical insurance was reasonably good, and I had enough money in savings that I could probably handle the costs that insurance wouldn't cover.

What worried and depressed me was how I was physically

going to manage taking care of myself immediately after the surgery. Remembering back to the previous spinal fusion, I was tormented with thoughts of the everyday practical problems of recuperating. I was divorced, my children were grown and gone, and I lived alone in a large, third-floor walk-up apartment. How in the world was I going to climb up and down those three flights of steel stairs? Carry the laundry to the laundromat? Drive the car? Buy groceries and carry them up to the apartment? Cook and clean?

There is no one, I thought, whom I dare talk to about these worries. Anybody will think I'm just feeling sorry for myself and whining, but that really isn't how I feel. It's just that I don't know how to manage the complications.

In the meantime, it was time to phone my mother and my friends, the Bittners, Wess Barrow, and Stanford Hall, and let them know where I was. Normally, I would be home from work by now, and if they called and I didn't answer the phone, they'd worry. I made the calls and played down the seriousness of the back problem. Tomorrow maybe I'd be less emotional about it and be able to talk better.

I put down the phone, alone again with my fears. "God, I need help. Pretty fast. I can't handle this."

Picking up the phone again, I dialed the church rectory and said to the gentle voice that answered, "Reverend Dillon, this is Lucy. Do you have a few minutes for me to talk with you?"

Chapter 2

A NORMAL RECOVERY: AWFUL

The spinal fusion was scheduled for two days later. During the waiting time I read, rested, and tried to make plans for what to do when I went home. And I tried to stop worrying.

At our school, we had a teacher from Los Alamos, Jeanne Scher, who taught classes for state-certified gifted children, and whenever they came to class carrying a load of worries, Jeanne said to them, "I want you to sit down someplace comfortable and close your eyes. Bring to your mind whatever it is that's troubling you the most. Now, in your imagination, pull out of your back pocket that black drawstring bag you keep. Open it up. Carefully place your worries in it and pull the string closed. Swing it around your head briskly and fling it over your shoulder as far as you can so that you won't ever see it again."

For two days of waiting, in my mind I flung black bags and tried to cast off my worries.

The spinal fusion was done by Dr. Schultz, Dr. Lloyd Hurley, and Dr. Gil Grady. There was nothing unexpected. Everything went as they had planned it.

The recovery from the back operation was a normal one: awful. I hated the terrible hurting, the loss of strength and energy, and being forced to make my chopped-up spine and hip bear my weight and walk!

I'm allergic to most painkillers, but sometimes it helps relieve the pain if I can get rid of some of my tension. Dr. Leo Buscaglia, the world-renowned psychologist, had come from Los Angeles a couple of times to work with guidance counselors, and I tried to recall his words in those seminars.

"I want you to form groups of five or six people and sit down on the floor in a circle. Now, I want you to lie down, still in a circle. Put out of your mind any everyday worries and concerns. Bring to your mind, instead, a scene which makes you happy and relaxed. Think about what you see, the colors and shapes, the sounds and smells, and who, if anyone, is with you. Submerge yourself totally in that vision and relax all your muscles while you enjoy it," he said.

Sometimes when I used that relaxation technique, I felt better. Always there was more of a feeling of peace.

It made me feel lots better, too, to remember the Buscaglia Hugs. What a cuddly bear he was!

Dr. Schultz, aware that I lived alone and that my apartment was on a third floor, felt that I should stay in the hospital a little longer than usual so that he could be sure everything was going well before I went home and was on my own. He arranged for the physical therapists to work with me twice a day to teach me the proper way to rise from the bed, how to use a walker, and how to turn around with the least amount of pain. Before I would go for a walk, even if it was only a dozen steps, the therapists fastened a heavy belt around my waist and held on to it to ensure against my falling. As my strength returned, our walks extended into the hall and, eventually, as far as the nurse's station, a hundred steps that seemed like a thousand.

The next assignment they gave me was to learn to climb stairs properly. They recommended to the doctor that I not be released from the hospital until I could climb up and down twenty-eight steps, the number of steps from the ground to my apartment. They started with a wooden set of two steps. "Up with your strong leg, down with your weak leg. Keep your weight supported by your stronger leg so that you don't have a collapse from weak muscles." Each day we added more steps. They worked, I tried and cried, and they encouraged me to try again.

As is normal, but I hadn't anticipated it, recovery didn't come about smoothly and evenly, each day better than the one before. Recovery seldom does, it seems. Instead, some days went well and others went badly. The bad days gave me a feeling of panic that something was wrong, and discouragement. I didn't want anything at all to go wrong. I wanted to get well, get out, and get back to work!

Many of my early apprehensions were unnecessary, it turned out. Why did I worry so much? I now wondered. Where was my faith? Didn't I know how good the doctors, nurses, and physical therapists were? Why hadn't I anticipated all the daily visits and help from Dr. Dillon and our other ministers at First United Methodist Church?

There were all my friends, too, more than I knew I had. My days were filled with their visits, phone calls, flowers, gifts, errands run for me, and homemade snacks from their kitchens.

Wess Barrow, my friend for more than thirty years, came to the hospital every day to find out what I might need, entertain me with funny and fascinating stories, and take care of the flowers and cards. If I needed some assistance from a nurse, Wess would draw herself to her full height of only five feet three in Gucci pumps, march to the nurses' station, and obtain their instant attention.

Daily visitors, too, were Beatrice and Barnett Bittner, who lived across the courtyard from me. During the summers, Bea and I met at the pool each morning to swim a mile, surrounded by trees, grass, and blossoms with hummingbirds whirring around them, underneath those brilliant New Mexico turquoise-blue skies. While we swam, Barnett took long, meditative walks in the gardens and parks.

When I first met Bea, she regularly swam at ten o'clock each morning, but she moved her time to seven after seeing me swim laps that early. She watched for a few minutes one morning, then turned to Barnett and said, "I'm not going to let a whippersnapper twenty years younger than I am outswim me," and changed her schedule to match mine.

Bea and Barnett had moved here from New York twelve years earlier. Barnett had successfully recovered from a massive heart attack and had retired from being a parole officer in Harlem.

You might expect a parole officer to be big and burly and tough, but not so. Barnett, whose college graduate work was at the Tulane School of Social Work, read, wrote, and spoke Hebrew, Yiddish, Russian, German, Spanish, and English. He lived in White Russia as a child and remembers his boyhood years reading *Uncle Tom's Cabin, The Prince and the Pauper,* and *The Adventures of Tom Sawyer* in Hebrew. Now, at age eighty-one, he wrote for *The Link,* a Jewish newspaper.

Bea had retired as the supervisor of the Welfare Department in Westchester County, New York, where she supervised nine offices. She had retired only in the sense that she was no longer on a salary, but stayed heavily involved in Albuquerque Jewish Community activities, social services, and charitable causes.

Bea and Barnett brought my mail to the hospital every day, took my gowns and other personal laundry home to wash and bring back, took care of my apartment, and stayed in touch with my mother to be sure she was all right and to assure her that I was all right, too.

Also helping me through this time was the Love of My Life, Stanford Hall. Stanford had been a friend of my family for more than forty years, and my own friend for ten. Fun, good-looking, and cheerful, Stanford brought his good humor to the Orthopedic Unit. You wouldn't know by looking at his casual style that this man was an attorney and a successful, powerful businessman throughout several states.

Stanford came to the hospital at 6:30 every morning and brought fresh doughnuts, hot coffee, and the morning newspaper. Under ordinary circumstances, we met for breakfast at a pancake house and then went for a brisk forty-minute walk. We had lots of fun talking about world events, business matters, our work, and our personal lives. "I don't see any reason to give up any more than we have to," he explained the first morning he came with breakfast.

During each day, he dropped in once or twice, or called, and then came back in the evening after work. His spirit and enthusiasm were infectious. I couldn't wait to get well and be able to go places and do things like we did before!

On the fifteenth day after the spinal fusion, when Dr. Schultz came in for his daily visit, he said, "The nurses and physical therapists tell me you're doing very well. We think you can safely go home anytime you want to. What do you think?"

"Yes, I agree. I'm doing well and I'd like to be in my own bed," I answered happily.

Dr. Schultz handed me a list of instructions and discussed them with me. "You're to continue to use the walker. You are *not* to stoop or bend down, reach above your shoulders, lift anything, drive a car, or sit or stand for more than a few minutes. I'll make arrangements through Home Health Care to have a nurse come to your apartment every day to look at your incision, take your vital signs, chart your progress, answer any questions you have, and arrange for any further medical help you might need. I want you to come see me at the office in two weeks, or sooner if you need to."

Throughout the two weeks I was in the hospital, I didn't admit to anyone, mostly out of misplaced pride, how worried I was about finding ways to take care of myself when I went home, but as it turned out, I didn't need to worry.

Dee Foster, a petite dynamo I worked with who came to the hospital frequently to see me, and who volunteered services like clipping the toenails I couldn't bend to reach, broke a surprise to me. "All your friends got together and arranged a program of care for you. Here's the plan, and you can tell me whether or not you like it, and what things you want to change. First, Stanford will come to your apartment every morning and prepare breakfast for the two of you and you can talk and read the paper before he goes to the office. The Bittners found a reliable housekeeper/aide that you can hire at a reasonable salary if you want her to come in for three hours every morning and help you take your shower and shampoo and help you get into your clothes. Remember, you won't be allowed to bend over, or to reach, and that includes getting dressed. She'll also straighten the apartment, freshen your bed—something you can't do now—wash the dishes and any laundry you might have, and prepare a light lunch for you."

This was beyond belief!

"Bea and Barnett will drop in during the afternoon to make sure you're fine and pick up your grocery list so they can buy your groceries and anything else you need. In the evenings, different friends will bring complete, nutritious meals that won't require any further preparation—no standing in the kitchen at a time when being on your feet for just three or four minutes, I know, is difficult."

Looking triumphant, she continued. "Your only work is to get well, so get to work!"

I was so moved! I couldn't believe that all these people had selflessly planned a complete program for my care. It was a lesson in the power of friendship. I felt that I'd never have enough opportunities to do for them all the things they were doing for me.

It brought to my mind the Theory of Good Deeds of my friend Agnes Moloney, from the Chicago area. While she was with the Cook County Hospital, she worked with a world-famous plastic surgeon to research and develop better, more modern treatments for serious burns and skin grafts for those burns. When war broke out, Agnes volunteered to be an army nurse and was stationed in England in a hospital that used the new techniques.

"The theory," Agnes once explained to me, "is that someone does a Good Deed for you, but for any of a number of reasons, you don't ever get an opportunity to return the Good Deed to that person. So, you do your Good Deed for some other person, a member of the World Bank of Good Deeds, whether or not he has ever done anything for you. That person then does a Good Deed for someone else who belongs to the bank. Very quickly the World Bank is filled with Good Deeds which it can lend out endlessly."

It looked to me as though the bank was well overfunded and I was so indebted that it would take me the rest of my life to restore the balance. I had so many reasons to get well!

Chapter 3

YOU MAY NEVER WALK AGAIN

By the time my back was well enough for me to return to work on a part-time basis, it was almost time for school to be out for the summer. Dr. Schultz talked with me about what I should do.

"Would the school system allow you to go back to work for two or three hours a day and then go home to rest for the remainder of the day?" Dr. Schultz asked. "Would you be able to do your job even though there were restrictions against reaching, lifting, carrying things, bending over, stooping down, standing, and sitting?"

Thinking carefully, I considered the requirements of my job and whether or not the school system made the kind of provisions that I'd need. "As far as I know, there's not any plan at the present time under which a counselor can work just a portion of the day and a substitute counselor can fill in for the rest of the time. It really wouldn't be practical either, given the nature of the work. As to doing my job when there are the restrictions such as you mention, I don't see how it would be possible. This isn't an eight-to-five office job. It's a busy, physically active, emotionally involving, day-and-night responsibility. After a full day in the office, there are conferences and meetings to attend at the central office, and children, parents, and teachers who phone me at night and on weekends at whatever time they need me," I replied, trying to relate a little bit about the kind of work I did.

"In that event," Dr. Schultz responded, "I think it would be better for you and better for your school if you didn't go back for the final few days of the term. Why don't you stay at home and finish healing now, let me remove the Orthofuse early in August, and by the middle of August you'll be well and you'll feel good. You'll be able to return to work at the beginning of the fall term in good health and not need any special concessions."

That made good sense to me, so I talked with the principal of the school and let him know that I wouldn't be returning this term and would need for the substitute counselor to stay until school was out for the summer.

Early in August, six months after the spinal fusion, Dr. Schultz removed the Orthofuse in outpatient surgery at the hospital, using a local anesthetic. For a few days my back was sore and tired, but that was the worst of it.

In mid-August I returned to my counseling job, but I felt bad. My back always ached. My hip hurt so much I could hardly move my leg forward to walk. It was really miserable to stand up for any length of time and sitting at meetings was an ordeal. It was hard to file any records in the lower drawers of the file cabinets and agonizing to move conference chairs and to carry test materials.

By late fall I was discouraged and depressed. How was I going to do a good job when I felt so bad? I went to Dr. Schultz for help.

Dr. Schultz made a new set of X rays and a new CT scan at the hospital. He carefully studied my gait, balance, and strength, tested how well I could bend forward, and checked to what degree I could do a straight leg raise. He asked questions about my daily activities and, indicating my lower back, asked, "Does this hurt when you sneeze or laugh?"

When all of the information was gathered, Dr. Schultz reviewed it with other doctors and then phoned me to come into his office. As he met me, there was a tightness in his jaws but a softness in his eyes that didn't correspond with the brisk matter-of-factness in his voice.

Something must be wrong, I thought.

"Do you see this vertebra?" he began, pointing to an X ray of the lower spine and counting aloud the vertebrae in my lower back. "That's an extra vertebra that most people don't have, and since you have an extra one, we'll be counting your vertebrae differently from other people's and you need to know that's why your records won't look like theirs. Here," he said, pointing to a joint in the lower spine, "is why you're having problems with your back. You don't have any disc between your lumbar-5 and lumbar-6 vertebrae. You also don't have any disc between your lumbar-6 and sacro-1 vertebra, the first vertebra below your lumbar-6."

That was impossible! It couldn't be! It doesn't happen. Maybe to somebody else, but not to me!

Yet, how familiar it seemed. Hadn't we just had this conversation a short while ago? As I had asked at that time, I asked again, "What do we do about it?" This time the question was edged with bitterness and the fierceness of a wounded, cornered animal.

"The appropriate treatment for these joints is the same as the treatment you had twice before for the same problem," Dr. Schultz replied with sadness. "You need spinal fusions at these levels."

Thoughts of again being betrayed and defeated by my back flashed through my mind. Was there any use in pursuing other options for treating my back if they weren't the answers to the problem? Should I see some other orthopedic surgeon for a second opinion? Would I just waste time and money duplicating the same tests, only to hear the same diagnosis? Dr. Schultz's reputation was of the highest, I knew that. Anyway, he'd already shown me the reports from the other doctors he'd consulted himself.

With resignation, but also with an overpowering need to get well, I asked, "Can you schedule the surgery to be done during the winter recess so that I won't be away from work so long?"

We scheduled the spinal fusions and the implant of another Orthofuse for December 23. It was a time for families and friends, Christmas trees and lights, parties and gifts, children and church and the Hanging of the Greens. Not back operations.

My spirits dropped lower and lower.

The surgery was performed by the same team as before, a team who knew my body and my reactions to trauma and stress. Recovery this time was harder and slower. My endocrine system, not a world-class system to begin with, went out of balance, and the dosages of medications I usually took no longer controlled my system. Also, I reacted to every painkiller we tried. My strength was slow to come back. The doctors kept me in the hospital longer this time than before, and when the annual meeting of our family's business corporation was held with the stockholders and Martin E. Threet, our corporate attorney, it was held in my hospital room in order for me to perform in my capacity as secretary-treasurer and member of the board of directors. The doctors, nurses, and aides considerately scheduled their activities around the meeting so as not to interrupt us.

Stanford resumed his schedule of coming to see me in the hospital several times a day. He looked after my apartment, watered the plants, brought things I needed from home, picked up my mail, and stayed in touch with my friends. They were coordinating their visits so that not too many people came to see me at the same time.

During a quiet evening when no other friends were in my room and doctors, nurses, and aides were working with their other patients, Stanford and I talked about our future and the good times we were going to have when my back got well again. He held my hand as we watched from the fourth-floor window the rich reds and golds of the desert sunset behind the purple volcanoes. It was a treasured moment filled with tender closeness.

"Stanford, I don't have the words to thank you for helping me through these bad times. I've been in the hospital at least thirty-two times in the past eight years and you've been with me during most of them. Anyone else would have left me long ago. What is it in your character that keeps you here? You have no obligation to me, no responsibility for my welfare. There's no legal tie or financial complication, and you're not a relative. I want more than anything to be with you always, but why is it that you stay?"

Stanford touched my face, caressed my shoulders, and

looked deeply into my eyes. "You need me. You've needed me from the beginning, and I love you," he murmured softly.

While I recuperated at home, the winter was cold and snowy and the nights were long and lonely. Pain from severed muscles, nerves, skin, and bones, and the weakness from the surgery, made it too difficult to bother to cook. Housework was restricted, so I couldn't keep my apartment as neat as I liked it to be. I'd never liked a house that was dirty or disorganized, and I fretted about it now. I wasn't allowed to drive the car yet, and I really didn't feel good enough to go out with friends, even as a passenger, so the apartment walls began to close in on me.

My life-style had always been busy. I'd been involved in a wide range of activities: business, church, social, and recreational. I wasn't used to being confined and inactive, and no matter how hard I tried to be a good sport about it and be patient, I wanted to be up and out doing things.

My friends continued to do everything they could to help me. They brought little meals, as before. They took out my trash. They talked to me about their jobs, their families, and their activities, and tried to keep me from thinking too much about myself.

Home Health Care resumed their services and sent a nurse to see me every day, and I rehired the housekeeper who had helped me before to come back and help again, but it bothered me a lot to be so dependent on other people for all of those things. My guilt deepened and so did my restlessness.

The days passed slowly. I hated the walker and the crutches, and I resented every restriction. Even worse, something strange was happening to my foot and leg and it was worrying me. Finally, one morning when Stanford came for breakfast, I took the risk of sounding like an alarmist and confided my fears.

"There seems to be something happening to my foot and lower leg," I said to him as we lingered over coffee. "Every day they get colder, and they're becoming numb. When I try to take a step, this foot doesn't bring itself forward the way it should. My ankle doesn't flex well, and I can hardly turn my foot from side to side. For the first few days I thought I was just imagining things, and then I decided it was just a phase of the healing process, but it keeps getting worse so fast that I don't know anymore what to think," I explained while I demonstrated the lack of movement in my foot and ankle. "Would you feel my foot and tell me if it feels cold to you, too?"

Stanford felt my foot and agreed that it was very cold. "Your foot is icy and has a bluish tone to it. You're right; you don't have much movement in your foot. Call Dr. Schultz this morning and make an appointment to see him. I'll call you at 9:30 to find out when it is and I'll come get you." He spoke calmly and matter-of-factly. He was certainly concerned and was going to make sure we did something to find out what was wrong, but he didn't do or say anything that would compound my anxiety.

Dr. Schultz asked me to come in at once and Stanford took me to his office. As I walked up the long hallway on crutches, Dr. Schultz watched. One foot moved forward as normally as could be expected after hip and back surgery, and the other foot dragged dead and useless behind me. "When did that happen? How can this be? Sit down here and let me look at that!" he exclaimed, anguish in his face.

The doctor ran sharp instruments up and down my left foot and leg and jabbed me with such sharp needles that he made me mad. "That hurts!" I yelped. Then he ran the same instruments over the right foot and lower leg. No feeling. Nothing. He tried to get a reflex. None. He ordered me to raise and lower my foot. No movement. "Turn your foot to the left. Point your toes as far to the left as you can." They didn't move. He felt the coldness in my right foot and tried to find a pulse. Gone.

Dr. Schultz's voice seemed too controlled, his face too serious, as he spoke with clipped words. "I don't know what's wrong, but I'm making an appointment for you to see a neurosurgeon immediately." He left the examining room briefly.

He soon returned and spoke brusquely. "I've talked with Dr. Mora and arranged for him to see you this afternoon. I've told him about the operations you've had and what's happening to your foot and leg. He'll examine you and call me to tell me what he finds out, and I'll call you at home just as soon as he lets me know what he thinks. His name is Federico Mora. He's an excellent neurosurgeon, and he's a very nice person. You'll like him." Dr. Schultz handed me an appointment card for Dr. Mora and helped me to the door.

Barely containing my emotions, I told Stanford what Dr. Schultz had said and gave him the time of the next appointment. He remained outwardly calm as he took me home to rest for a couple of hours before we went to see Dr. Mora.

At Dr. Mora's office the nurse assisted me to a seat. The neurosurgeon questioned me about the problem I was having. When had I first noticed it? What change in my foot had I detected first? How rapidly did it seem to be changing? What other operations had I had before the most recent spinal fusion? Did I have any health conditions? Did I take any medications?

We went into the examining room. The nurse helped me onto the examining table and stood my crutches in the corner.

"I'm going to press several instruments against both of your feet and legs. I want you to tell me what you feel," Dr. Mora said as he raked my left foot with something that felt like a set of razor blades and then jabbed me with sharp needles. I jumped and winced and glared at him in anger. Next, he used the same instruments on the right foot.

"What do you feel now?" he asked.

"All I can feel is that you're pressing something against my foot, but I don't feel any other sensation," I answered. "This foot feels dead compared to my left foot."

"I want to see how much movement you have in both of your feet, so follow my directions carefully," Dr. Mora said.

He ran through the same tests Dr. Schultz had done and a number of others before he concluded his examination. Dr. Mora, neatly slender, a very elegant Latin, spoke with a soft and romantic accent. "Mrs. Dobkins," he began, "I don't know the reason for it happening, but something is compressing the nerves in your right foot and leg. There is apparently something which shouldn't be there pressing against them. The only way I can find out what's causing the compression is to be able to look at the nerves themselves. You're going to need a nerve root decompression."

Panicked at the idea of more surgery, I asked, "What's a nerve root decompression? How do you do it? How bad is it?"

"A nerve root decompression is an operation done through the back. You'll go into the hospital and have a general anesthetic. I'll ask Dr. Schultz and Dr. Hurley to assist me, and in the surgery we'll open your recent back incision and carefully move all of the muscles out of the way again. Then we'll take apart all of the slivers of bone used to fuse your vertebrae so that we can get down to your spine and see the nerves, trace them, and find whatever it is that's pressing against them. After we release them we'll put your fusions back together again."

I cringed and shuddered, wondering how I could possibly go through that all over again. But Dr. Mora wasn't finished with what he had to say.

"We'll have to do this operation immediately. And I can't promise you that a nerve root decompression will do you any good. You might never walk again," he concluded.

My hands flew uncontrolled to cover my face and hide the shock and terror and torrent of tears that poured down my face.

I had no words to say.

Chapter 4

TED'S CAREER IS RUINED, POOR GUY

For the third time in a year I made all the personal and job arrangements needed for another hospitalization and told my family and friends I was going to have a back operation. Again. I had barely finished filing insurance forms for the last surgery and now I had to phone each insurance company, tell them what was going to happen, and request new sets of claim forms. Were insurance claims always a hassle to everyone, I wondered, and then you have to wait, wait, wait for the benefits to be determined and paid? But what would I do without them?

Stanford had helped me pack for the hospital so many times that he really could have done it by himself. What I needed packed the most, however, was a suitcase full of optimism.

Every time I'd been at St. Joseph's, Bea and Barnett had visited me every day. They were in such a habit of turning off the freeway at that exit that they continued to turn there even when I wasn't in the hospital. "It's going to be easy for you to get back in the habit," I told them. "I don't like to be a problem to you, but I hope you'll come see me."

The staff in the Orthopedic Unit were surprised to see me return and they felt bad about the back operation to be performed the next day. They tried hard to ease my apprehension. The nurses were gentle when they did the preliminary prepping

49

that night, and they were especially careful as they completed the prepping the following morning. "We wish you the best of luck, and we promise you'll have the best of care," they said as the escort wheeled me to the operating room.

The orthopedic surgeons and neurosurgeons opened my back through the same incision made earlier and examined the fusions that had been done so recently. They were amazed and distressed, when they were finally able to clear everything out of the way and examine the spine, to discover a tiny chip of bone slipped behind the spinal cord out of sight pressing against the nerve, permanently damaging it and causing my foot drop. They freed the nerve, cleaned the area, and made some small repairs before putting the fusions back together and closing the incision.

For the second year, spring was a time of confinement and recuperation. My floppy, lifeless foot was now strapped into a fiberglass form that had been molded to my foot and leg and fitted with Velcro straps to fasten it around my leg. My flat, ugly shoes were a size and a half larger than normal in order to accommodate the form.

My other equipment included a wheelchair and a walker to use in the apartment. At a later time I'd go outdoors with them and eventually I'd graduate to Canadian crutches, the lightweight aluminum crutches that reach only to the elbow, and clip around your forearms.

The weeks dragged into months of living with my limitations and not feeling good. Stanford helped me pass the time. On Saturdays we made popcorn and watched Ted Kitchel, my cousin, play forward on the Indiana University basketball team that Bobby Knight coached. The team played powerfully, and Ted, his brilliant moves scouted by other teams, was said to be a first-choice draft for the NBA at the conclusion of Indiana's twenty-six-game season. My uncle Edwin phoned my mother from Indiana every weekend and shared his pride in Ted.

Suddenly, just five minutes into a game with only two games left in the season, Ted asked to be taken out of the game. The arena crowd, television viewers, fans around the country, and the national press clamored for news. Was Ted hurt? What happened to him?

The next day Uncle Edwin telephoned Mom and told her Ted was in the hospital for a spinal fusion.

I asked Ted to tell me everything that happened, but that was much later, after he was well.

"When I began playing basketball for Indiana University," Ted began, "I'd already played throughout high school, so I was strong and physically fit from running several miles a day, going to workouts, practicing ball, and playing in the games. College basketball practice was more strenuous, though, and I began to have a lot of pain in one hip. When I did straight-leg exercises and bent to touch my toes, the pain worsened. When I sat in classes, the calf of my leg ached a lot and I kept moving around in my chair all the time.

"I had no knowledge about back problems and didn't know what was the matter, but the trainer figured that some ultrasound and heat treatments would help. The coach sent me to an orthopedic surgeon, but he didn't know what was wrong. They brought in a neurosurgeon to examine me."

"'Lie down flat on your back and raise this leg as far up as you can,' he told me.

"I could only lift my leg about twelve inches off the examining table.

"'Pull your toes and foot toward you and hold them while I try to pull them down,' the neurosurgeon said.

"My foot had no resistance against the pressure.

"The neurosurgeon directed, 'Now point your toes and your foot away from your body and hold them firmly while I try to bend them toward you.'

"Again, no resistance, no muscle strength, no control. The doctors ran further tests and said the disc at lumbar-4 was ruptured and fragments were probably pushing on the sciatic nerve, causing the pain in my hip and back."

Ted continued. "They kept me in bed, lying on my side, blocked with pillows for two weeks and the doctor gave me muscle relaxants. I got well enough to go back to basketball practice, but I found I couldn't play in the games.

"The neurosurgeon decided to do microsurgery to clean out the fragments of disc and fuse the vertebrae. He hadn't ever performed a spinal fusion on an athlete and Indiana University hadn't had an athlete who needed one, so no one knew what to anticipate or how soon I could play basketball again. The university now got their experience, though, first with me and then with another guy, a great player who had the same thing happen to him a couple of weeks later. He got well enough after his fusion to go on and play professional basketball for the Golden State Warriors in San Francisco and the Los Angeles Clippers.

"Thankfully, I was in excellent physical condition and I was back to normal in two or three weeks."

"What happened to you after that?" I asked, amazed at such a rapid recovery.

"I played basketball for Indiana University for four years and didn't miss another game. The neurosurgeon gave me regular follow-ups, and I got along without any problems. Then, one week at the end of my senior year, I didn't feel right. I told my trainer and he said, 'Don't worry about it. I'll take care of it.' I figured he knew better than I did, so I went ahead to a practice session."

"Was that smart?" I asked.

"Well, I was one of the captains and I didn't want to complain or quit. But during practice I made an offensive move and felt something in my back explode. I finished the practice anyway in a lot of pain and went on to the game that night."

Ted explained, "When you play basketball, you kick your legs out in front of you, but in this game I couldn't do it. It stretched the sciatic nerve too much. I played five minutes and couldn't go on, so I asked to be taken out of the game. I didn't have any feeling below my knee and I was afraid I'd injure it or break it by not being able to feel.

"Till the game was over, I lay on a bench in the locker room with my legs drawn up to try to relieve the pain. We all flew home the next day and I went into the hospital for a myelogram and other tests. It turned out that the disc at lumbar-5 had ruptured, and three days later I had another spinal fusion."

I could sympathize.

"This operation was harder. The doctor was cutting through scar tissue. Afterwards, the pain was worse and I asked for pain shots every three hours on the hour. Nevertheless, they had me up and walking within eighteen hours and, you won't believe it, but three nights later my doctor told me he wanted me to go to the game my team was playing. So, my mom and dad made a bed for me in the van and we drove to the game. During the game I sat on the bench with the other players and after the game I gave a press conference. By then I was drained totally!"

"It's unbelievable that you could be in such good physical condition that you could do that!" I exclaimed. "How did everything go after that?"

"I had a tougher, slower comeback this time, and more pain. The doctor said more surgery might be necessary if additional problems developed.

"After graduation I was picked to play professional basketball in Trieste, Italy, for good pay. During the first two weeks, and I was playing well, the team owners took me to five or six of the finest specialists in Italy and Yugoslavia to have my back evaluated. The owners needed assurance that if they put me under contract for $75,000 to $100,000 a year I'd be able to play out my contract. They finally decided they couldn't take the chance."

"What did you do?"

"The Milwaukee Bucks drafted me for the NBA. I played well during practice sessions and I passed the physical with flying colors, but one night at a practice game the doctor called me to the sidelines.

"'I'm not going to okay you to play professional ball. I don't think your back can take league play and league players. I think it's more important that you be able to walk around, play with your kids, and play golf when you're forty than to play basketball for a year or two in the National Basketball Association,' he told me."

Ted's mother, Barbara, had told me it was hard for Ted to give up his career: the games, the travel, the big money. As a mother, she was relieved that Ted wouldn't be participating in a physical sport any longer, but she did sympathize with him.

I asked Ted how he felt about the loss of his career.

"Well, that's just the way it goes. Life's kinda funny. But I can't be bitter. Basketball gave me a free education, let me travel and play ball all over the world, and I'm very fortunate."

Stanford and I talked about how disappointing it must have

been for Ted to have to give up what he was trained to do and the promise of financial success, and then have to find a new direction for his life. "Ted's career is ruined. Poor guy! How does a person handle that? That's something I'd hate to have to deal with," I said.

Continuing, I philosophized, "Don't you think it's even harder for a man to have a back problem than for a woman? If a woman says she can't lift something, men are always ready to help her and they think nothing of it. Society is used to regarding women as weaker than men, but when a man has a bad back and can't lift something, he's extremely reluctant to ask someone else to lift anything for him, and if he does, people sometimes regard him with skepticism and suspicion. Does he really have a bad back or is he trying to get out of the job? is what they ask themselves."

"There's truth in that," Stanford replied. "The trouble with having a back problem is that you don't wear any bandages or casts that everyone can see and know you're hurt."

He was so right!

Chapter 5

AND NOW WHAT?

The doctor had cautioned me that I might not walk again, and so far there hadn't been anything to indicate any improvement. If that was the case, now what? Maybe I'd better think about my own career. How was I going to continue my profession if I couldn't do the job? And how about my personal life? How could all of this be happening to me anyway? Me! The girl from the Western high desert and the Rio Grande Valley. The girl who likes to ride horses, backpack in the mountains, hike down the Grand Canyon, climb the face of the 10,000-foot Sandia Mountains, scuba dive, deep-sea fish, water-ski, play tennis, bowl, dance, and work in the yard. What was I going to do about the rest of my life if things didn't get better?

Day after day, night after night, the anger and grief overwhelmed me. It just wasn't right! It wasn't fair! I'd spent my whole life unselfishly giving of myself to other people. I'd never knowingly been wicked, and I didn't deserve this! Like Job in the Bible, I dared to question God's sense of justice and I protested against it violently. I cried out, as did Job, "Why me?"

On a sunny Saturday morning when the trees and shrubs were bright with purple, pink, yellow, and red spring blossoms, Stanford came over and said, "Let's go for a ride. I have a store grand opening today and I need to be there. I want you to see the store with me."

He helped me into the wheelchair, cheerily pushed me out to

the parking lot, placed me in the station wagon, and folded the wheelchair into the back.

This was my first excursion out into public since I'd developed the foot drop and had the surgery to free the nerve. "I'm really embarrassed to be seen this way," I complained, referring to my foot that wouldn't work, the form encasing it, and the wheelchair. "I don't want anyone to see me or think I'm a cripple, and I don't want anyone to pity me."

"Just forget there's anything wrong. Look at it this way: you're going shopping and so are the other people in the store. That's all anybody cares about."

We went into the new and crowded store filled with colorful, bright new merchandise and I forced myself to concentrate on admiring the store and doing my shopping, rather than thinking about how conspicuous I was with my wheelchair. Just as I was beginning to forget myself, who should we bump into, shopping in the same aisle, but my good, longtime friend Dee. I was so fond of Dee that I had deliberately evaded telling her how things were going for me, and I'd put her off when she'd asked to come see me. That was a mistake—a selfish one.

Dee's expression was a play of shock and anguish and then quick composure.

"Lucy! When did you start shopping with a limousine and a driver? Stanford, are you available to take me shopping at, say, three this afternoon? Will you drive a limo for me, too?"

She made a determined effort to treat my personal distress lightly and joke with Stanford about my condition, but I was ashamed of how I'd treated her and I could see that she was deeply upset at finding out about me in this accidental manner.

Later Dee would tell me, "After you and Stanford were out of sight in another aisle, I rushed to the check-out counter and dropped all my items there and didn't even wait to check out. It was all I could do to get home before I cried. I cried a lot that day. And prayed."

People often say to someone who is sick or hurt, "Well, it could be worse! Look at so-and-so and his problems." They said that to me all the time, too, and it always made me mad. I wanted to yell at them, "You just don't know anything about what it's like!" Sure, I knew other people had bigger troubles than I had; I'd been in the counseling profession and in hospitals enough to see that. But I had all I could handle and that's what counted for me at that moment. Maybe, when things got better, I'd have the mental energy to sympathize again, but not now.

Pride made me want to be strong, healthy, and whole, not crippled, and I wanted to hide my damaged body from the world. Stanford knew, however, that I needed the stimulation of being with other people, going places, seeing interesting sights, and doing activities we both liked. More and more frequently he took me in the wheelchair out for breakfast or lunch, or for a drive around town inspecting his shopping centers and other developments. He talked about real-estate transactions that were in the works, banking activities, real-estate development plans, and news of a broader range. He didn't allow any time for me to think about myself while we were together, and when we got home after each excursion he'd say, "Okay, here you are. It's time for your jazzercise. I'll leave you to your workout," and leave.

Dr. Schultz had prescribed exercises, though they weren't jazzercise, to do at home. One of them was utterly boring and useless. His directions were, "Sit down with a rolled-up towel under your bare foot. Take the ends of the towel in your hands. Pull your foot up toward you and let it down. Do this several times a day and try to reintroduce movement to the nerves. Make them remember what they're supposed to do."

Faithfully I did what Dr. Schultz said to do several times during the day and at night, but it was dumb and ridiculous. My foot and toes were dead and wouldn't respond in any way. It was a waste of my time. (Oh? So what else did I have to do with my time?)

Then, late one evening, sitting in front of the TV and resenting pulling on my towel and foot, I felt the smallest movement in one toe. It was so unexpected that I was shocked, and then I disbelieved it when I recognized what it might mean. I tried again to move my toes and foot and this time I watched and paid close attention. Once more that one toe twitched.

At that moment hope reentered my life. Movement! At least

some of it *was* going to return! I was certain of it. I *was* going to walk again!

I was ecstatic! Insane, actually. I laughed and yelled and cried and wanted to run outside and show the whole world what I could do with one toe. "Oh, God, thank you! Thank you! Thank you!" I shouted deliriously.

Early the next morning I phoned Dr. Schultz and told him about the toe responding. "Let's start you in a physical therapy program here at the clinic," he said, "and see how much the nerve will regenerate. Can you come in at one o'clock today?"

Jo Ann Swinson and Niame, the physical and massage therapists at the clinic, tested the strength and amount of movement in each foot and leg and brought out some electrical equipment.

"This machine with the cords and meters is a high-voltage electrical stimulation machine. These knobs here are for you to control the frequency and strength of electric current we're going to conduct to your body," Jo Ann said, indicating the knobs on the front of the machine. "This is an electrode and pad to carry the current. They'll be attached to a spot on your buttock and stimulate the nerve that we want to regenerate. This other electrode and pad will be attached to your foot. The jolts of electricity won't hurt you. You yourself will regulate the current to be as strong as is comfortable. We'll give you a series of mild shocks which will cause your buttock and foot to jump. We'll increase the amount of time and the strength of the shocks over the next several weeks. The purpose is to agitate and stimulate the nerve to regenerate and to remember how it's supposed to work and help bring the muscles back into use. It also increases the blood circulation. We'll do some muscle-strengthening exercises with you to build up your foot and leg, too."

Jo Ann connected the electrodes and turned on the current very slightly. "Now," she said, "you turn it up as high as is comfortable for you. If it becomes uncomfortable, turn it back down. If you have any questions or problems, I'll be right here in the room. Just call me." She drew the curtain closed.

Jo Ann treated my leg and foot five days a week for many weeks and gradually more and more sensation and control began to return, enough that I could control my foot sufficiently to get rid of the Canadian crutches and just wear the brace.

The second Orthofuse was still implanted in my back and anyone could actually feel it under my skin just below the ribs. If I leaned against a chair it hurt and sometimes it bothered me to lie on it in bed. Maybe it was increasing the speed of healing; for certain it was entertaining my friends. They had fun pretending to be horrified that there were electric wires inside my back. "Don't go into the swimming pool. You'll electrocute somebody!" "She walks through the courtyard and all the apartments light up!" were some of their irreverent remarks. They'd walk through the apartment humming "You Light Up My Life." I was glad they thought it was funny. I needed some laughs.

After the Orthofuse had been implanted for nearly six months, Dr. Schultz had me check into Day Surgery at St. Joseph's so he could remove it. There was nothing to it, even though he had to leave the wires, too imbedded in tissue to pull loose. They wouldn't cause any problems in any event, so it was of no concern to either of us. In fact, I speculated that maybe a little wire with some string and bubble gum would help hold me together.

Another summer passed. It was August and time for me to return to work. Finally! But how? I was out of the wheelchair, walker, and crutches, but I still wore the leg brace, had considerable lower-back pain, walked with a lurch, lacked energy and strength, couldn't lift or carry things, couldn't bend down to the lower file drawers, and couldn't stand up or sit down for any length of time.

I'd been on medical leave for two years and, although my position was held for me, I was not on salary. My sick leave had been used up long ago and I had no other income. My savings account was draining rapidly. I wanted to work and I needed to work.

"You'll need to get a letter from your doctor releasing you to resume working," the personnel director said when I told him I wanted to start the fall term, trusting that I would feel better as time went on.

I phoned Dr. Schultz and told him what was required before I would be accepted back on the payroll.

"Come see me tomorrow and bring a copy of your job description," he said.

Dr. Schultz made a new and thorough examination, the X-ray technician, Forrest Fouch, made a new series of X rays of my spine, and the doctor took me into his office to look at them and talk.

"Your X rays are fine. Do you see the white, fluffy cloudiness around your fusions? That's new bone gathering. Can you see where the sharp, dark edges of the plugs of bone are now blending in with older bone? Look at the alignment of these vertebrae. Technically you're beautiful!" Dr. Schultz said proudly as he pointed to each area of the spine. "But the patient still feels bad and the patient wants to go to work anyway. Did you bring a copy of your job description? Good. Let's look at it."

I handed him the papers and talked about my work. "The job of a guidance counselor in a junior high school includes personal conferences with students, parents, and teachers, and all counselors know the conferences are often highly emotional and not the kind of conference you can terminate when a pre-established time is up. You have to stay actively involved and see it through. Precise timing is required in doing psychological evaluations and other testing, and we don't do anything that will interrupt or distract the client.

"Group conferences require that chairs and tables be set up in any of several offices, meaning we move furniture. Presentations to parents, teachers, and administrators are given standing up, usually with audiovisual aids like projectors and screens and printed materials, all of which have to be carried to and from the meeting. When we take cases to court, we sometimes sit all day long on a hard bench, not getting up to stretch or walk around. Student registration requires standing in front of classes all day long for several weeks, carrying boxes of registration materials not only to the classes in our own building, but also to the classes in five other schools which will send us their students next term."

"What other regular responsibilities are there?" Dr. Schultz asked.

"We don't have any secretarial help, so we take care of student records ourselves, pull files from the drawers, high and low, and replace them when we're finished. Counselors assist with supervising students, too. We climb up the wooden bleachers to sit with students during assemblies, stand in the halls during passing time between classes, and stand in the cafeteria to supervise students during lunch."

"What hours do you work?"

"Actually, I work more than my contract requires. Generally I'm in the building at seven o'clock every morning and I don't leave until after four o'clock, and then I go to counselor meetings and task-force committees which are formulating policies for a system to evaluate all the employees in the district and we have about six thousand employees. I take work home, too, and spend several hours each night working on my case files."

"Do you have to do these extra things and work the number of hours you're working?" Dr. Schultz asked.

"No. If I just did the minimum job, I might not have to, except that I've heard there's a proposal to change the hours this next term and require that counselors work ten hours a day."

Dr. Schultz continued to study the job description. He got up and left the room for a few minutes. When he returned, he sat down across the desk from me, looked at me very directly, and stated, "You'll never be able to return to the kind of work you were doing."

My mouth fell open. I blinked in disbelief, not sure I'd heard him correctly.

"Not do what I was doing? Not be a counselor?" My mind whirled. "Does that mean I can't go back to teaching either? Or to administration?" I asked haltingly, shaking my head and swallowing hard.

"Yes, it does mean that. Your back physically cannot do what those jobs require."

Well! That was an outcome that had only barely crossed my mind because of Ted Kitchel, but I hadn't ever given it any real thought. I didn't want to accept it as the truth, but deep in my heart I knew that Dr. Schultz was right.

God, when am I ever going to get out of this mess? I wondered.

"Stanford, can you come over? I need someone to talk to and I'd like for it to be you. Yes, as soon as you can. Thanks," I said into the phone.

During the few minutes it took Stanford to drive to my apartment, I sorted out my thoughts. Stanford was my confidant, but there were things I had never wanted to tell him about myself. They were things I'd never told anyone, actually. I wanted people to think I was strong enough to handle anything that came my way and I did my best to hide my warts and weaknesses. I intended now to ask Stanford to help me decide what to do with my life, since I was losing the old one, and he'd be able to advise me better if he knew more about me.

With trepidation at revealing myself, as well as trust in Stanford's judgment and discretion, I answered the knock at the door.

Chapter 6

A NEW BEGINNING

If it's stormy in the north, I look only toward the south.

MARY K. ZARTMAN

Stanford came in from the warm summer night and embraced me.

"Thanks so much for coming over. Come in and have a cup of coffee. Dr. Schultz gave me some unexpected news today that I don't know how to handle, and I really need your help. I'd like to tell you some things about myself that I haven't ever told you, except for a few small things from time to time. Now I have to take inventory of myself and if you'll let me tell you what I've done in the past, maybe you can help me decide what to do in the future. Would you listen to me for a while and give me your advice?" I asked.

"Of course! I hoped you'd tell me more about yourself and I was just waiting until you were ready. I want to know everything about you and, if I can be of help, I will be," Stanford replied sincerely as we took our coffee to the living room.

"I was married for twenty-one years," I began. "I thought it was a pretty good marriage. We had a lot in common, our work was similar, our goals seemed to be the same, we had two good boys, a nice house with a pool and shady yards, vacations in Europe, England, Canada, Alaska, and Mexico, a couple of boats and a camper, and a little money in the bank. I happily looked forward to growing old water-skiing into the sunset.

"Then one Sunday afternoon my husband returned from visiting his parents nearby, and abruptly said, standing in the hallway, 'I'm leaving. I've made arrangements to live with my parents.'

"Incredulous, sure I hadn't heard right, I said, 'What do you mean? What are you talking about?'

"'I'm moving out,' he answered tersely.

"'That's crazy! Why? What's wrong? What've I done?' I demanded to know.

"'You haven't done anything. For some reason that I don't understand I just have to hurt you. You deserve a chance to find someone better than I am,' he said, and with that remark he turned, walked out the front door, and never returned.

"He refused any communication with our sons, Rusty and Terry, and he wouldn't talk with me. He didn't even explain to his parents why he'd moved in with them. None of us understood him and none of us knew what to do.

"A few days later I answered the phone and a voice I didn't recognize told me in a secretive manner that my husband was going to marry a friend of mine as soon as he could get a divorce, and he wanted the divorce as fast as possible. I couldn't understand how I could have missed the clues or how I could have been so blind. I was shattered. In empty rooms I railed against the unfairness of it and grieved at what had happened to our life together. I expressed my desolation in a poem I called, 'I Need a New Life, God.'" I showed a copy to Stanford:

I NEED A NEW LIFE, GOD

I need a new life, God.
The old one's swept away.
One hour the sun was rising,
There was rhythm to the sea;
Then the ocean wind blew shreds of mist
Between my love and me.

The oleanders and hibiscus
Bloomed their brilliant, fiery hue,
While hummingbirds and sea gulls
Shared the fantasy in view.

I closed my eyes for but a moment
Standing on the shore,
And when the waves came crashing in
My love was there no more.

"We did get a divorce and he did marry my friend and, then a short time later, he divorced her and married her secretary. It was devastating. Any hope of happiness became a dead coal. What good was it to try to be a good wife and mother? What was the use of investing everything in a long-term relationship only to see it spat on?

"The divorce settlement left me with the house and the mortgage, the usual kinds of family bills, two nearly grown sons to help through college and to establish in business and to set up in housekeeping, on one-third the income as before. At about the same time, my health became a concern and each doctor who ran tests sent me up the line to a higher specialist. Finally the diagnoses began to come in: Addison's disease and hypothyroidism were the first problems to be identified and from then on the other functions of my endocrine system began to topple like dominoes on a shaky table.

"During the time I'd been married, my social life was built around other couples and families. Suddenly that life was gone. I was now A Single Woman. I didn't fit. There were only a few people left in my support group and I thought I didn't dare burden them with my problems or I might alienate them and not have anyone at all.

"Fortunately my family was a rock. My parents, my brothers, Dave and Jim, and my sister, Helen, understood how devastated I was and telephoned from their happy homes in other states to encourage me. Helen especially seemed to have ESP and always knew when my spirits were the lowest and I needed someone the most.

"My family and I had belonged to the same Methodist church since 1934, when we moved here from the snows of Indiana, and that was the church where I'd met and married my husband. Our sons were baptized and brought up there. After the divorce our minister and members of the church did all they could to help me accept and cope with the breakup of our marriage.

"Thankfully I had a good job. I was a guidance counselor in a new school not far from home and I worked with children from the first through the ninth grade. I was actively involved in developing several exciting new programs and field-testing them, including special-education programs for various levels of disabilities and programs for gifted children. When I was at work I was totally involved in what I was doing and I didn't think about my personal life. It was therapeutic for me to focus outward.

"Following the divorce, I went through changes of emotions like clouds in the wind: hysteria, despair, guilt, shame, anger, and loneliness. There was a period of time when I was probably psychotic and needed help, but the cost of therapy, and my pride, kept me from getting it. Also my field of work was mental health, I reasoned. As much experience as I had in helping other people solve their problems, I ought to be able to solve my own. That was a bad mistake. I should have talked with a psychologist and dealt with the problems outright.

"Eventually my emotions leveled out and I could think more clearly. I made two resolutions for the future: one, I wouldn't allow this bad experience to make me bitter against men or friends; and two, I would increase my professional credentials and therefore my income and security.

"My sons enrolled in college and so did I. I already held a bachelor of science degree in elementary education and a master of arts degree in guidance and counseling and in administration. The State Department of Education had certified me to teach all subjects in grades one through eight and six subjects in grade nine. I also held a state certificate in guidance and counseling for kindergarten through the ninth grade and I'd already been accepted into a Ph.D. program in administration, so my advisor developed a schedule of evening and summer classes which would let me complete the program while I worked.

"The way I arranged my schedule was this. Early mornings from five o'clock to eight were for breakfast with my sons and straightening the house and watering the yards. During the day I worked, of course. In the late afternoons I helped the boys with their homework and paper route and prepared dinner. After dinner they studied and I went to class at the university.

The late night was the time for me to study and write papers. Weekends meant laundry, housework, yard work, cleaning the pool, servicing the cars, and doing things with and for the boys. On Sunday afternoons I went to the university library to do research in the stacks."

Throughout this time Stanford was totally attentive. Not knowing how he was feeling about what I was telling him and wanting to give him a break, I asked, "Would you like some more coffee? What I'm telling you is heavy stuff, baring my soul, and it's probably even harder for you to have to listen than it is for me to tell you. May I fill your cup?"

"I'll get it. Do you want cream and sweetener in yours? Don't even think about it being hard for me to listen. I'm glad to finally know more about you," he answered, getting up to go to the kitchen.

With fresh, hot coffee I resumed. "During that time my father was killed and my mother was left alone at the age of seventy-five in our big family home on the farm. My brother Dave and his family came home from Kuala Lumpur, Malaysia, managed the business, and took care of our mother for a year, but when his leave of absence ended he returned to his profession in genetics research and as a university professor and department chairman.

"It became my responsibility to look after the business: lease the crops and watch the harvesting; lease the rental houses and rental corrals; oversee the care and maintenance of the properties, machinery, and equipment; do the accounting; and handle the family's corporation business with our CPAs and attorneys.

"Increasingly Mom needed more care. She had strokes, falls, and serious illnesses rather often, but she didn't want anyone to live with her and she didn't want to leave her own home to live someplace else. I kept myself on call, day and night. I phoned her frequently and if she didn't answer her phone when I thought she should, I made a speedy drive from the far side of town out to the valley. Four times when I got there she was almost dead. The risk became too great to continue the way we were and I tried to think of something we could do that would allow her to remain where she wanted to live, but at the same time give her more safety.

"Bea Bittner, also concerned, told me about a program called Life Line sponsored by the Heights General Hospital in town and I made an appointment to talk with the director. He showed me an electronic device which they could connect to my mother's telephone. 'If she has a medical emergency and needs help, all she has to do is press a button and the device automatically dials the switchboard at the hospital. The operator immediately dispatches an ambulance and a staff to go to her assistance. An additional piece of electronic equipment is this small pendant which your mother can wear on a cord around her neck. If she needs help when she isn't within reach of the telephone itself, all she has to do is press the center of the pendant and the telephone connection to the hospital is made and an ambulance is dispatched.'

"'With this device,' I said to him, 'my mother can be less anxious about going into the basement or taking long walks out through the yards and fields she loves. It will give all of us more peace of mind.'

"I talked it over with Mom and we had the system installed.

"Finally I received my certification in administration from the state. My course work for the Ph.D. was about finished, too, and there wasn't much more to do in order to receive my degree except to take a year's leave of absence to do my residency and write the dissertation. However, that was no longer feasible for me.

"My sons finished their schooling, entered careers, and got married. After the boys left, I sold the house and moved into this apartment, where there'd be less maintenance, no empty rooms, and no ghosts of what used to be.

"I changed from a school in a high socioeconomic community to a school which had three poverty pockets and the highest rate of crime in the city and I expanded my experience.

"I was elected president of the New Mexico Personnel and Guidance Association, which is our state professional organization, and developed a major convention for counselors, special-education directors, and administrators to move forward in developing statewide programs for gifted children. I brought Dr. Leif Fearn, the authority on programs for the gifted, from San Diego State University to guide us.

"During the winter months I worked with the New Mexico state legislature to enact tougher laws regarding child abuse. I made presentations regionally and nationally in regard to special-education and counseling programs I helped develop and test, and the articles I wrote on counseling and special education were published in professional journals. I participated in field testing for UCLA their model for leading adult discussion groups and participated in Dr. William Glasser's 'Schools Without Failure.'

"More and more frequently I was asked to serve on steering committees and task forces for the district and I kept a high profile.

"The superintendent appointed me to be the summer-school principal for two junior high schools, now called middle schools, an assignment widely regarded as a proving ground for administrative candidates, and afterwards my name was placed on three independent lists for promotion to year-round administration of a school of my own. I was just waiting for the next vacancy to occur at the end of the term.

"My life was finally running smoothly again and I didn't hold any bitterness about the price it cost. I had developed a new, large collection of interesting friends, I was becoming fairly sound financially, and my long-range career goals were apparently only weeks away from being achieved.

"It took me twelve years to get where I am, twelve really hard years, but I didn't let anything distract me from what I set out to do. You came into my life and brought me the first real happiness I've known in a long time, and you haven't ever said or done anything to interfere with what I was trying to accomplish. Did you ever wonder why I seemed so driven?"

Stanford just smiled.

"From the moment I hurt my back at school, I've been worrying that the superintendent would move my name to the bottom of the promotion lists and all those years of work would be for nothing.

"Today Dr. Schultz studied my job description and talked with me about it and it looks as if my efforts to succeed and gain some security were futile regardless. He said I can't ever go back to the kind of work I was doing. I have training and work experience in other fields, too, like government, banking, oil, farming, leasing, the travel industry, and fashion, but I can't go back to any of them either with my back the way it is.

"Now I'm at an age that many employers won't be interested in me, but I'm too young to just sit around. Listening to all of this objectively, what do you think I should do?" I asked.

Stanford had sat very still and listened carefully to everything I said. Now he stood up and silently walked around the room, pausing now and then to consider. At last he turned to me, put out his arms, and brought me into them for a loving hug.

"Let's consider in two ways what you've said. I watched your face while you talked and I saw when you were teary. The nervous activity with your hands and the bouncing of your foot told me some more about sensitive areas of what you said. Let's set that part of the conversation aside until another time when we can talk about that all by itself. For now let's deal with the immediate issue of what you can do with your life."

Taking my hand in his he guided me to the sofa and began to talk. "It looks to me as though you need to look into retirement first. You have more than enough years of service to be eligible and your pension can provide some basic income.

"Then why don't you talk with Dr. Schultz about his projection of the amount of time you still need in order to complete the healing process and find out what he anticipates the eventual condition of your back will be.

"Finally," he said, choosing his words carefully, "it looks as though you need to own your own business. You need to choose work that's interesting and challenging and can provide a secure financial future, but one that also allows you to determine your own work schedule, to take rests when you need them, to do the tasks you're physically able to do, and to hire people to do the things you can't."

This was becoming exciting! A new beginning! "All right, what do you think the business should be?" I asked.

"For a long time you've talked about wanting to own a lingerie store. Why don't you begin some serious planning and run your feasibility studies? We can make some trips into other states and work our way up the West Coast to study other stores and interview owners. I happen to be in a position to help you find a good site. You can design the store and develop your business plan while I locate the site and negotiate for it. We can prepare your pro forma together."

We talked into the night, exploring ideas, discarding unworkable ones and listing the good ones that merited further thought and conversation. The more we planned, the more enthusiastic we became.

It looked as though there might be a productive future for me after all and it would be great fun to plan it with Stanford!

Chapter 7

BAD BACK:
COPING FOR LIFE

"What can you tell me about my back and foot? Are they going to get well? How long is it going to take?" I asked Dr. Schultz.

Stroking his distinguished-looking beard, rocking from heel to toe, arms folded across his chest, Dr. Schultz regarded me carefully. "You're making new plans for your life? All right, the first thing you need to do is accept the fact that you have a bad back and you'll be coping for life. You'll probably always have a high level of chronic pain that you'll just have to learn to live with, but there should be a little less pain than there is right now. A certain amount of it will ease off as you gain more muscle strength.

"From studying your X rays," he went on, waving a large manila envelope filled with negatives, "we can see that your entire lower back is fused so solidly that almost nothing can happen to it. About the only problem that can come up is if a vertebra above the fused area becomes bad."

"That sounds positive enough to me. I can take a lot of pain and it doesn't scare me. Are there ways to speed up the recovery and to stay healthy from now on?" I asked, encouraged.

"Sure. Continue the things you're doing. Restrict your physical activities and avoid anything that stresses and strains or jolts your back. Learn when you need to sit or lie down. Keep doing the exercises the physical therapist showed you and resume swimming regularly, but don't use a butterfly stroke or a back-stroke. Eat a nutritious, balanced diet and stick with the regimen of medications, vitamins, and minerals your endocrinologist developed with you. Continue taking your injections of estrogen to control your osteoporosis and keep your weight where it is."

"How about my foot?"

Dr. Schultz knelt down, removed my homely shoe, and studied the brace that cradled my foot and leg. "You have probably seen about all the nerve regeneration you're ever going to see in that foot. It's improved enough that it will control the muscles as soon as you build more strength in them. Over the next few weeks you can gradually increase your foot exercises and work your way out of the brace. Start by going a few minutes each day without it and increase the time according to your muscle strength. Don't walk too far and get overly tired and be very careful not to fall. Don't jolt that spine!"

"When can I wear dressy shoes?" I asked, knowing I was pushing my privileges.

"In good time," Dr. Schultz replied with a smile, unruffled.

The next appointment was at the school district's Employee Benefits Office to inquire about retirement. The supervisor knew my name and history and was aware that I had been on medical leave for quite a long time.

"If you're considering retiring, let's work up a benefit form right now and I can explain to you how to apply, what amount of benefit you're eligible for, the tax benefits, and the health-insurance conversion procedure with the increased premium you'll have to pay," she said.

On her computer she pulled up my work history of service and salary and made the calculations of percentage of salary that retirement is based upon, the number of years of service, and my age. She then calculated the pension figure I could expect to receive.

"You do need to know that if you want your retirement to be effective this year, the deadline to apply is today and we'll have to call the capitol in Santa Fe to enter your application effective today and then mail the paperwork to them tomorrow," the supervisor said.

Thinking carefully and deliberately, I answered, "All right. Let's file the application today." I was certain that it was what I should do, but nevertheless there was a hard lump in my throat knowing that I was closing the door on twenty-six years of work I loved and believed in. Of all the ways to try to make a contribution to society, the fields of education and mental health were two of the best. I would miss the work, the families, and the professionals I associated with.

My formal retirement was concluded with letters of appreciation from the superintendent and the Board of Education, a silver bowl, Waterford crystal, and a round of retirement dinner parties. An era of my life was over. It was time to move ahead.

For a long time I'd talked about owning a lingerie and fur store, but that was to be ten or twelve years in the future. All of a sudden the future was now and there was plenty to think about and do if I decided to move in that direction.

A mutual friend of Stanford's and mine was a successful businessman who had in the past listened to my ambitions about owning the store.

"What made you want to own a lingerie store?" our friend asked one day at lunch with Stanford and me.

"When I was a little child during the war, good fabric and nice underclothes were hard to get, so my mother used to save the prettiest, softest muslins with pretty printed flower designs from sacks of flour to make my sister's and my little dresses and underclothes from them.

"One summer, however, Mom ran out of the pretty flour sacks and just used a regular flour sack to make my underpants.

"On a warm day when Helen and I were up in the tops of our big cherry trees picking cherries to can, one of our hired men walked under the tree, looked up at my bottom, and snickered. Then in a loud voice that everyone around could hear he said, 'Oh! Pillsbury!'

"I was so humiliated that I determined that when I grew up I was going to have the finest, most beautiful lingerie I could find."

He and Stanford laughed, especially at seeing that I still felt insulted.

Then our friend said, "When you decide you want the store, let me know. I want to be your silent partner. You can plan it and design it, do the buying, select the staff, manage the business, and consider it yours. I'll be available for any business consultations you might want, and I'll partially back you financially, but my name is not to be mentioned. Does that interest you?"

"Does it ever! This is my chance, probably the last chance I'll ever have, to build a financial future, and it will be so much fun! Let's do it! You won't be sorry. I *have* had a store before, you know."

The men, surprised, asked in chorus, "When was that?"

"When I was about five. My family had just moved to Albuquerque and my father bought a new farm, so I wanted a new store on the sunny side of the house under the shade of the big trees in the yard. I set up my counters, stocked the shelves with groceries from my mother's cupboards, and hired my boyfriend, also five, to help me run the store. We figured our probable sales and had grand ideas about how we were going to spend all the money we were going to make. Our venture looked really good until I painted *STORE* in big, black letters on the side of the house. After that neither the store nor I survived very well."

I assured them, "Now that I know more about landlord restrictions regarding signage, I'll do a lot better."

Our friend and I drew up a contract and I began the plans. Stanford started searching for a site with high visibility, maximum traffic flow, and easy access in an established shopping area.

It wasn't very long until I felt good enough to travel. Stanford and I studied the major lingerie stores, department stores, and shopping malls in the surrounding states and on the West Coast, studied manufacturers' products and prices, learned what kinds of merchandise had the fastest turnover, and interviewed store owners, accountants, lawyers, and bankers about the lingerie business. We did a market survey, which told us who our buyers would be and the kind of merchandise and service they would want. I spent a number of exciting days in the Los Angeles Mart, the California Gift Show, and Brack Center, met with manufacturers, designers, and sales representatives, and learned how to buy merchandise in such a way as to have new stock arrive every day, the right items in the right quantities and sizes.

In the meantime, Stanford tentatively selected a site. My silent partner and I both liked it, so Stanford negotiated a contract. I designed the store, drew it and the furniture and fixtures to scale, and took the plans to Peter Grivas, the interior designer who'd done some other regional stores so tastefully.

Peter's dark Greek eyes flashed with interest and growing excitement in the possibilities for the store and he began to draw. "I can design all of your furniture, the cash desks, shelves, storage rooms, workrooms, everything, and we can build it all right here," he said, waving to the manufacturing area of the plant.

While Peter worked on designing and manufacturing the furniture and fixtures, I designed a large *U*-shaped desk for my office and contracted with a cabinetmaker to build it. Finished, it was a beautiful piece of workmanship. The single unit functioned as a personal desk with a typing area that included a filing system. With half a dozen upholstered swivel chairs on the two outer sides of the unit, it was our conference table for staff meetings and conferences with businessmen and sales representatives.

It was time to select a name for the store and we deliberated over it. We wanted one that would be somewhat intimate because of all the sleepwear for men and women and decided to call the store "Lucy's Pillowtalk." We commissioned Dennis Magdich, the Chicago artist now living in Santa Fe, to design our logo, a beautiful, long-legged girl in a lacy teddy, and we contracted with manufacturers to design and produce our business cards, stationery, and all of our bags, boxes, and ribbons.

I developed a detailed business plan, printed and bound it in gray suede, presented silver-monogrammed copies to my silent partner, Stanford, and the vice-president of the bank we chose, and opened a commercial account. My silent partner made a substantial initial deposit and I tapped all of my remaining resources, including an inheritance I'd kept separate from regular savings, and deposited my contribution.

The plan was for the store to be a medium-sized lingerie store, but also much more. We planned twenty-three departments to include intimate apparel, loungewear, hostess-wear, silks, furs, gifts, custom-designed fine jewelry, custom-blended fragrances for men and women, and a men's department with robes, pajamas, slippers, warm-up suits, sweaters, cashmere-lined gloves, briefs, and fine toiletries.

Bea and Barnett, sharing the excitement of the venture and the elation of a new beginning for me, cautioned me. "Just don't push yourself. We know you're having fun and you want to build something for your future, but nothing is worth getting sick over it!"

"I agree with you completely. I'm following all the instructions and taking good care of myself," I assured them. "Everything is moving into place right on schedule, and I'm learning to live with the pain too. The real test will be next week when I go to market in Dallas. There'll be a lot of walking and long hours, but I plan to limit myself as much as I can. Don't worry about me."

The first trip to the Women's Apparel Mart, Menswear Mart, World Trade Center, and Dallas Trade Mart was an astounding, fabulous experience, beginning with dinner at Loew's Anatole Hotel and a gorgeous room.

"Let me tell you what it's like!" I said excitedly to Stanford when he picked me up at the airport upon my return. "Imagine going to the biggest shopping mall in this state and stacking six more malls on top of it. Add scads of escalators and elevators, restaurants on every floor, and showrooms filled with the most beautiful merchandise that 15,000 manufacturers can present: clothing and shoes, furs, jewelry, bags, gifts, and a lot more. And, that's just part of only one of the buildings! Picture 12,000 to 16,000 buyers in the Mart, each one looking Dallas-chic. Then visualize buyers, including me, at the end of a twelve-hour day, slowly walking down the last corridor, shoulders slumped from carrying our briefcases, order books, appointment calendars, and aspirins, with our alligator pumps in our hands because there is positively no other place we can bear to wear them. I love it!"

Happy, though tired and aching after the flight, I went home to a long, hot bubble bath and bed, content that this job was the one I could handle in spite of my back. When had I ever had so much fun?

Our store held its champagne grand opening the day after Thanksgiving, the biggest shopping day of the year, just in time for the holiday shopping season. My partner and Stanford watched the crowds of customers and were optimistic. "The merchandise is excellent, the men and women on the staff are well trained to give the best service, and the crowds are heavy. I think she has a winner," my partner said. And Stanford agreed.

A few weeks later Stanford asked, "Now that the store is open and running smoothly, when do you plan to go to market again?"

"Early January will be the next trip and I have a schedule right here for you. These are the market dates for the rest of the year. I'll go to Dallas, New York, San Francisco, Los Angeles, and Las Vegas to buy merchandise. There'll be a buying trip every six to eight weeks. Can you go with me?"

"No. I have my own work to do. This is yours. Go enjoy it," he said.

One trip was not so much fun though. On the second day of the Dallas Market, I came down with stomach flu, which made me too sick to leave my room at the Wyndham Hotel and keep my appointments at the Mart and also too sick to catch an early flight home. The manager of the hotel was ready to send for an ambulance to take me to the hospital, but I didn't want to go to a hospital away from home and alone. He called the house doctor, but when the doctor found out my medical history he said he wouldn't treat me without talking with my Albuquerque endocrinologist. So I phoned my home doctor myself. He phoned a pharmacy in Dallas and ordered the medications I needed and the hotel staff brought them to me.

During the third day of nausea I thought I was well enough to be able to sip a little soup and I called room service. The moment the fragrance of the soup filled the room, I got sick all over again. Gagging, I stumbled my way to the door and set the food tray outside in the hall, and guess what! The door closed behind me, locked of course. There I was in the elegant hall at the top of that beautiful pink marble hotel with nothing on except a black lace nightie and a short marabou wrap over my shoulders.

After I walked barefooted up and down the hall knocking on doors, one door finally opened and a girl peeked out with wide eyes, wondering what this strange woman wanted. Desperately I said, "I've locked myself out of my room. Could you call the front desk, please, and ask them to send a security person with a key to let me in?" Not very eagerly she said she would.

I went back to my doorway and huddled up to it as closely as I could, trying to be invisible until someone came with a key. Finally I heard the elevator door around the corner open and close and I stepped out of my doorway with a huge smile of appreciation—only to look into the eyes of a guest of the hotel in a dark-blue, three-piece suit, with a wide grin and long, lingering look over his shoulder as he passed on up the hall.

The security man arrived right behind the guest and asked me, shivering from chilliness not fear, if I'd been frightened. "No," I said. "I wasn't frightened. Just so embarrassed!"

The security man looked at me good-humoredly and answered, "Don't be. This happens all the time. That's why I love my job!"

My partner and I regularly consulted about the store, including the personnel. "You should set the work schedules for your staff and yourself so that you can work whatever hours are best for your health and, if you get too tired or hurt too much, go home for an hour and lie down," he suggested. "Keep enough employees to cover the work when you leave for a while and also hire a manager to take over some of the work that you do."

In theory what he said was good. It just didn't work. When you own your own business, I quickly learned, you're likely to work *all* the hours, your own and your employees', too, whenever someone calls in sick.

Following my partner's suggestion, we appointed Tom Wingfield, an employee who had been with us since we opened the store, as manager. Tom, tall and slender with a handsome head of graying hair, had retired from a military career and tours of duty all around the world. After his retirement he attended the Robert O. Anderson School of Business at the University of New Mexico and received his degree in business shortly before he came to work for us. He had been an officer with significant responsibility, he'd had experience in the retail business, and he was absolutely reliable. He also had the most gracious manners you could ever want and our customers were quite taken with him, sometimes to his discomfort. Tom welcomed the advancement, and the opportunity to learn more about this particular business and to have more responsibility in running it.

Working in the store, I found that it was hard to be on my feet hour after hour in the sales area, even though that was the part of the store I liked best. Our customers became my friends and confided to me their love lives, their romantic successes and failures, and their sincere efforts to improve their relationships. They talked with me about their most secret personal thoughts and asked for my advice. I listened to the wives of prominent pillars of the community wish their husbands would wear the silk pajamas and robes they bought for them, and then listened to the husbands who said they wanted to burn their wives' old flannel pajamas and get them to wear the silk gowns and negligees they bought for them. I seemed to be a bedroom counselor they could talk to and trust not to repeat the conversations. What a delightful change from child-abuse cases!

In order to protect my health, I learned to vary my activities: an hour or more in the sales area, then some desk work and phone calls in the office, then go run the business errands and do the banking, continuously using different muscle groups to keep me from getting so tired that the hurting became too great to stand.

Our staff did the physical work: lifting the boxes of merchandise brought by UPS, unpacking the shipments, sewing our labels into the clothing and steaming it, and carrying the new merchandise to the sales area.

"Even with all the accommodations I'm making and the work the staff is doing, there are times when I have to go into the office, close the doors, and lie down on the carpet until the pain in my back lets up," I confided to Bea one evening when she expressed concern that I didn't look well. "It hurts my back if I bend even slightly to arrange the jewelry in the display cases. If I move a garment rack even a few inches, my back and hip hurt terribly until I can get to bed at night. I'm having headaches, pains in my tummy, pains in my chest, and difficulty breathing. At night I'm exhausted and I fall asleep quickly, but the aching is so bad in my back and hip that I can't stay asleep."

Bea gave me her "I knew it" frown but didn't say anything.

"I'm even forgetting things for no reason, important details. In fact, last week something happened that really did alarm me. I was at the mall where I've gone for twenty years and suddenly I didn't know what city I was in or which mall it was, and I didn't know how to find the exit to go to my car. I was so disoriented that someone had to lead me to an exit." I hated to tell Bea these things; she was already so worried about me.

"You get yourself to the doctor and find out what's going on. And stop working so hard! The store will run without you!" she scolded.

The endocrinologist I went to, suspecting that my system was out of balance again, ran batteries of tests and sent me to Anna Kaseman Hospital for a brain scan and chest X ray. There was nothing out of the ordinary in the results.

"If there's nothing showing up, why do I feel so bad?" I asked, puzzled. "Except for how I feel, I'm having the happiest time of my life."

"I don't know what's wrong," the doctor answered, equally mystified. "I want you to cut back your work hours, get more rest, and call me in a week."

During all the years of knowing Stanford, he'd phoned me at 5:20 every day to say good morning and we decided where to meet for breakfast at 6:00. After breakfast we walked briskly for forty minutes and talked. We embraced and kissed goodbye and each went to work. My hip, however, now made every step so painful that I could hardly put weight on it, yet I stubbornly refused to give in to it or to say anything that would jeopardize these mornings that meant so much to both of us.

My personal life was going well. My mother was aging, but her health was greatly improved. In fact, after some deaths in the family, my mother detailed to me what kind of funeral she wanted when her time came and she asked about her will, her finances, and her crypt at the mausoleum.

I answered all of her questions and, satisfied with the answers, she switched gears and asked me, "What provisions have you made for your own death?"

"I have a will, too," I began, startled, "and the will designates that my body will be cremated and the ashes will be scattered over my favorite bays in the Sea of Cortez."

My mother, eighty-six, looked at me in shock and exclaimed,

"Then we won't ever be able to see you again!" as though she'd be around forever herself.

I laughed, hugged her tiny, fragile shoulders, and said, "Mom, that's not the way it's supposed to work. I'm going to be here a lot longer than you are and you'll see all you want of me. I plan to look after you as long as you want me to and you don't need to worry about anything."

Lucy's Pillowtalk was growing and, as we went into our third year, we were projected to gross $325,000 in sales. This would be our year really to become established. It was exciting and I was so very grateful for having been given this opportunity.

"My entire life has turned around," I said to Stanford as we lay in front of the fireplace. "I am so happy that you've stayed with me through all those bad times and helped me get to this point! I'm having a wonderful time and I love you for helping make it possible."

He snuggled me a little closer in the glow from the flames and we contentedly listened to the crackle of the fire.

My life had turned around, it was true, except that any movement of my hip had become so excruciating that I could hardly walk. I limped like a cripple: one of those "physically challenged" people. That was not my image of myself. Fewer hours and easier work at the store didn't make any difference at all.

Schultz hasn't seen me for a long time, I thought to myself. Maybe I need a hip transplant like my mother had. She recovered very well, even at her age, so it wouldn't be too bad for me, this much younger. I called for an appointment.

Dr. Schultz entered the examining room, slapped his forehead, and said gruffly, "I don't want to see you. You're a nice lady and I like you fine, but I don't want to know if something else is wrong with you."

I just smiled and said hello.

"All right, go ahead and tell me," he said resignedly. "What's wrong?"

Knowing that he sincerely cared about me, I wasn't offended by his rejection, and I went ahead and described the hip pain, constant lower-back ache, sharp, jabbing pains if I turned or twisted, headaches, forgetfulness and disorientation, poor balance, fatigue, chest congestion, and difficulty breathing.

Dr. Schultz made an examination and was noncommittal as

he summoned Forrest for X rays. "This lady needs some pictures of her lower back," he said and dictated the views he wanted.

Forrest left and closed the door behind him. Critical that Dr. Schultz hadn't gotten to the problem at all, I objected. "You didn't order any X rays of my hip, did you? How can you tell what's wrong with it just by looking at my lower back?"

Dr. Schultz looked at me with the most pained eyes I've ever seen, put his hand on my shoulder, and solemnly, quietly said, "There's nothing wrong with your hip. It's your back."

Stunned and speechless I joined Forrest in the X-ray lab. It took his help to climb up on the X-ray table. It hurt to move or to lie flat, to turn from side to side, and to climb down when we were finished. Every movement was painful.

When the X rays were developed, Dr. Schultz studied them, took me to the lighted glass on his wall, and hung the negatives for me to view. "Do you see this line running all the way across your fusion on both sides of your spine? That's a nonunion, a break. God only knows why, but your fusion never healed after the operations three years ago and every time you move, you pull and pound the vertebrae and the nerves. I also think you have spinal stenosis again. There appears to be blockage of the nerve that runs to your foot.

"I want you to see Dr. Mora, the neurosurgeon who did your nerve root decompression the other time, and find out what he thinks. He's already acquainted with your back, but I'll talk with him before you see him and review your medical history with him." He shuffled some papers on his desk. "I want you to go to St. Joseph Hospital for a bone scan and a CT scan. I'll have a consultation with the doctors there rather than just getting their usual written report. I want to know everything they find and get their opinions as to what we should do. I think you're going to need another spinal fusion and another nerve root decompression and, if that's right, maybe we can do them both in one procedure and make it easier for you."

Dr. Schultz was clearly as distressed as I was. Regarded as the premier orthopedic surgeon in town, he was also a very kind, sensitive, gentle man. This was as bad for him as it was for me, I knew.

As I left the doctor's office, tears streamed down my face. I got into my car and pounded the steering wheel in rage and frustration. I sped recklessly to a nearby secluded parking lot, turned off the motor, and sat there, screaming into the cold winter darkness, "No! No! No! No! Not anymore! I can't do this anymore!"

Chapter 8

LIFE, HOW CAN YOU BE SO PERVERSE?

Lacking the composure to talk to anyone about the new X rays but obligated to let Stanford and my partner know there was a problem, I told them only that Dr. Schultz had seen me and was sending me to St. Joseph's for further tests.

Dr. Schultz talked with me and said, "I feel bad about the timing, but I'm scheduled to leave in a week for Africa and I'll be gone a month. Before I leave let's get your studies completed at the hospital, let Dr. Mora examine you, decide what we'll need to do, and set a schedule."

How disappointing that he was leaving—leaving when I needed him!

"Usually," he continued, "I order a CT scan, a bone scan, and a myelogram, but let's not do the myelogram on you right now. There's a possibility you'll react to the dye and feel more discomfort than you already feel. I'll have Harriet make your appointments." Harriet Gerardo was his nurse, kind and efficient, who meticulously studied every patient's chart, knew what the problems were, and followed up on any further studies that needed to be made.

"As soon as we have all that information and Dr. Mora sees you, I'll talk with you again," he concluded.

At 7:30 the next morning I checked into the Radiology Unit

as an outpatient. Déjà vu: same nurses, same technicians. "We're so sorry you're having problems again! What's happening?" they asked, concerned.

They began their work of adjusting knobs, dials, and cameras, positioned me properly on the X-ray table, and prepared to make their technologically advanced X rays. Every position on the hard, flat, X-ray table was so painful and difficult that the technicians kept telling me I must tell the doctor how serious the pain was. They finished the CT scan and gave me the directions for tomorrow's bone scan. "You're finished for today but we want you back at 7:30 tomorrow morning. We'll give you an injection of radioactive material at that time and send you away to do whatever you want to do for three hours. Then you'll return to Radiology for more X rays."

I understood. I'd done this before.

"While we do the bone scan, you'll be able to watch on the monitors here and here," the technician said, pointing to the computer screens, "the dye travel through the pathways throughout your entire body. That test will enable the radiologist to detect whether there is any cancer or other 'hot spot' disease in your bones."

The following day the bone scan was completed and a syringe of spinal fluid was drawn from my spinal cord to test for any disease such as cancer in the spine.

The tests were painless. It was just the climbing up and down from the table, turning from side to side, and lying with my back and legs flat against the table that hurt so much and made me feel too bad to go to the store later. All I wanted to do was go home and go to bed.

The radiologist and Dr. Schultz studied the X rays and tests together and drew their conclusions. Dr. Schultz phoned me to come to his office for the results.

"There's no evidence of disease and that's good. But you do have a non-union of your spinal fusion and, if Dr. Mora confirms that you have spinal stenosis, we suggest that we do both procedures in one operation. We can schedule it for the second day after I get back from Africa. That will make it March 28th," he said, studying his desk calendar.

"Who would assist you in the operation?" I asked. "What's the procedure?"

"I'd want Dr. Hurley as assistant orthopedic surgeon, Dr. Mora as neurosurgeon, and Dr. Grady as general surgeon. Rosemary Harrison is always my surgical nurse and she's done all of your operations. They've all worked with your back and they know your health conditions.

"The procedure," he continued, "would begin by turning you on your face while we make an incision in your back where we made all the others and Dr. Mora will do whatever he has to do in order to free your nerve from the thing that's pressing on it. It could be bony overgrowth at a nerve opening from the spine and, if it is, he'll have to scrape it off. When he's finished decompressing the nerve, we'll turn you over on your back and do an anterior spinal fusion. That's done through your tummy."

"What can I expect afterwards?"

"You'll only be in the hospital for a couple of weeks, but I won't want you to work for a year in order to give your back a chance to heal solidly."

"A year! But my store . . . !"

"You're not going to be able to work in your store: the long hours, the desk work, all the standing and selling, and the pressures of owning that kind of a business. I know it's not in your nature to lie back and let the store run itself or to turn it over to employees. The store might mean a lot to you, but your back is more important."

This wasn't the time for me to dwell on it. Later, though, I'd think about it a lot.

Dr. Schultz phoned Dr. Mora while I waited, reviewed my health history, and told him he believed I had spinal stenosis and needed a neurological evaluation. Dr. Mora said he wasn't able to schedule me immediately, but he'd be able to evaluate me shortly after Dr. Schultz left on his trip. Dr. Schultz penciled onto his desk calendar the date of March 28 for surgery, pending Dr. Mora's evaluation.

"Lucy, I'm sorry to leave you at this time. Take it easy and I'll see you as soon as I get back," Dr. Schultz said.

"I will. Have a great time, and bring me a baby elephant with a strong back."

There couldn't be any more delay in telling Stanford and my partner what was happening. They had a large interest in me, personally and in business, and all our plans were about to change. If I couldn't work for a year, how could we keep the store? My partner hadn't ever been interested in running it himself; he had enough businesses of his own. Our manager was good but when he and I had divided up the work, I had only given him certain areas of responsibility and I'd maintained the other areas for myself. The finances were mine, personnel and advertising were mine, and I was the buyer. Tom could manage everything else well but there wasn't enough time left to teach him my jobs. A store like this really needed two of us anyway.

I'm cornered, I thought. What am I going to do? If my partner thinks we should close the store, how will I tell the staff? There'll be eight households without a job and those eight men and women are like family to me.

I asked my partner and Stanford if they would meet with me. "There's something I have to tell you, but first I need to explain some things that have been happening," I began when we met. I wasn't going to like this meeting at all.

"Since the last back operations, I've had sympathetic dystrophy in my right foot. I haven't told you or anyone else that I've been going to St. Joseph Hospital as a day surgery patient for a number of weeks. I've had about thirteen epidural blocks, nerve blocks as they're called, to try to get control over the sympathetic dystrophy."

"What's sympathetic dystrophy?" Stanford wanted to know.

"The entire mechanism of sympathetic dystrophy isn't understood medically. It results from a change in the sympathetic nerve system after some kind of trauma, major or minor, on a reflex basis. For example, a mechanic lying under a bus gets his legs run over and the nerves are damaged. A painter is on a high scaffold that collapses and crashes to the ground, seriously injuring him. Or too many back operations can cause it," I explained.

"How does it act?' my partner asked.

"In my case it makes my toes unbearably sensitive and my foot icy cold. If I stub my toe against a chair, it hurts like a major injury. There isn't much feeling in the rest of my foot, though, and if I lose a slipper in the house, I don't know the difference unless I happen to look down and see that I'm barefooted. I go back through the house, room by room, till I find it. Because of the sensitivity in my toes, shoes and stockings are uncomfortable. Also, during many nights there are jolts of electricity that zap my foot so hard that they're too excruciating to stand. I can't bear to have covers over those toes and I often sleep with my foot outside them."

"What are the nerve blocks supposed to do?" they wanted to know.

"Sometimes injections of steroids and anesthetics into the nerve will allow warmth to return to the foot and will lessen the sensitivity in the toes. With some patients one injection is all it takes and for others it takes more. In my case, the anesthesiologist, Dr. Rashi Jo, determined that the effect was so minimal and lasted such a short time that he shouldn't give any more of the injections. It's an ordeal anyway and sometimes I react to the medication and go into convulsions. Dr. Jo always stays beside me until the period of possible reaction is past and he's certain that I'm fine. I wanted the nerve blocks to help me but they didn't, so that's that."

Stanford was looking uneasy. "How are the injections given?" he asked.

"The way it works is I check into Day Surgery and the nurses take my vital signs and weight and fill out their intake forms, change me into a gown, and give me a curtained bed. The anesthesiologist arranges me in a curled-up position on my side, creating as much arch in my back and as much space between the vertebrae as possible. Next, he injects a local anesthetic between the two vertebrae where the nerve to my foot is. In a few minutes he injects a long needle into my spine and shoots steroids and anesthetic into my spine."

"Why haven't you said anything?" they asked, perturbed.

"I have a philosophy about illness. The less you say about it, the less you think about it and the less you draw attention to it from other people. My approach to illness is to ignore it till it goes away; if it doesn't go away, work harder and forget about it and don't make a big deal out of it."

Stanford, not at all pleased, glared at me. "Do you really think that's a good philosophy?" he asked coldly. "Do you honestly believe you shouldn't tell me your toes hurt too much for anything to touch them? That the rest of your foot is so dead that you can't even feel your slipper? That you've been in the hospital thirteen times in the last few weeks? Is that a philosophy you'd like for me to adopt? Should I not have let you know when I was in Intensive Care from a heart attack? Or when I had insulin reactions? Or just about died from sunstroke in the desert?"

Scorched by his burning anger and contrite that I'd carried things too far, I shrank.

"But that's not the only reason we're here, is it?" my partner asked. "You have more to tell us."

"Yes, I do, and I can hardly tell you this. I'm not in very good control of myself," I said haltingly, shifting my aching back and hip. "Dr. Schultz made some new studies of my back and he'll have me see Dr. Mora for confirmation. It looks as if I have a broken spinal fusion and also spinal stenosis. I'm scheduled for surgery five weeks from now and I'll probably be in the hospital for a couple of weeks."

Neither man moved. I took a deep breath, bit my lips, clenched my jaws tightly, and continued. "Dr. Schultz said I'm not to do work of any kind for a year in order to give my back a chance to heal and he said I shouldn't ever return to working in the store." There. It was done.

Dead silence. What were they thinking?

My partner gently said, "Call a meeting of the staff and tell them we're selling the store because of health reasons and we'll make sure everyone gets a good letter of reference and a good job."

Stanford looked at me across the desk and said, "Anytime you want someone to help you look for your slippers, just give me a call and I'll be there."

The store was my pride, my livelihood, my entertainment, my recreation and social life, and it allowed me the excitement of traveling. It wouldn't anymore, though. We drew up plans to sell it.

I met with the staff for a half-hour of poignant emotions ranging from empathy for me to their own concerns for themselves. I asked them to try to stay with us to the end, assured them of excellent letters of reference, and promised to help them find new jobs. They expressed their desire to do anything that would help, whether it meant more work, longer hours, or more responsibility, anything to relieve my anxieties about leaving. They vowed to support Tom when he took over.

I made lists of everything I needed to do for the store during the next five weeks. The list included writing letters to the 300 businesses, manufacturers, and banks we did business with around the country to tell them we were selling the store. As soon as the first letters were delivered, the long-distance calls, letters, and cards began to arrive.

"Lucy, this is Simon Katz in New York. We just got your letter. My God, girl, what's wrong?" A brief explanation. Silence on the line. "Lucy, I'm so sorry. I love you and I'll be praying for you. Get well fast and open another Pillowtalk."

Myrna Farnum and Edris March, the owners of Fame Time in Los Angeles, phoned. "Lucy, we're bringing you a get-well card. We'll be there Thursday."

Jim Brodie and Art Coley, owners of Designer Showcase in Dallas, called. "We'll miss you at the market. We'll call you again when you have your surgery. God bless you."

The calls continued. How could I walk away from the reps and designers, manufacturing presidents and credit managers, models and actors who'd become such good friends? I wondered unhappily.

There were personal arrangements to take care of, too. I phoned Marilyn Goodsell, the manager of the retirement center where my mother now lived. "Marilyn, this is Mary Zartman's daughter. I'm going into the hospital for a back operation and won't be able to look in on her for a while, so I want to give you the names and numbers of some friends you can always reach in case of emergency."

I phoned Helen, Jim, and Dave and asked them to phone Mom especially often for a while and make sure she had whatever she needed. I phoned my kids.

Stanford, concerned at the turn of events, gave me encouragement, suggestions, and help to get everything ready.

Even though I cut back the number of hours I worked and I didn't spend any more time in the sales area, the back and hip pain worsened. At night I couldn't sleep on my back, it hurt so much, and it hurt just as much to lie on my sides. So consequently, I hardly slept at all. Nor could I sit comfortably. Walking was also difficult and five minutes of standing in line at the grocery checkout were enough to make me faint.

My peculiar-acting foot was familiar to me by now, though not the least bit welcome. Alarmingly, however, between Friday night and Saturday morning, I became aware that I was rapidly losing strength and control in my ankle and foot. My foot wouldn't pick up normally, nor would it point forward or set itself down properly. My ankle kept turning to the side, flopping almost. It felt the same way that it had when the foot drop was coming on three years ago.

What's going on? What's happening to my muscle control? I don't like this! My mind was getting ugly images and I was uneasy.

With a feeling of urgency I phoned Dr. Schultz's answering service at noon on Saturday. "I'm sorry, but Dr. Schultz is not on call this weekend. Dr. George Dixon is taking his calls. Would you like for me to page him?" asked the operator.

Dr. Dixon had sewn up my badly hurt son years before and I was happy to have him available.

He returned my call and, after hearing the background, said, "I think you should admit yourself into the hospital today and stay there until Dr. Schultz can make an evaluation on Monday. You should also call your neurosurgeon and let him know what's happening. I'll call you again tomorrow to find out how you're doing."

I phoned Dr. Mora's service and asked to have him paged. "I'm sorry, but Dr. Mora has recently had surgery and won't be seeing patients for several weeks. Would you like to talk to his partner, Dr. Ralph Kaplan?"

The call back from Dr. Kaplan was prompt. I introduced myself, told him the background of what was happening, and what Dr. Schultz and Dr. Mora were planning.

"I don't think you need to go to the hospital yet, but you should go to bed now and stay there. Come into my office on Monday and let me see you," he said.

On Monday I went to Dr. Kaplan's office. A bearded, solid-looking man with piercing eyes, he made no small talk; he went straight from "Have a seat" to "What's the problem?" My first impression was that he was cold and gruff and didn't like my complicating his busy schedule, not that I blamed him. My experience later was that he was a very interested, attentive, alert doctor, sensitive to his patients and entirely sympathetic.

Dr. Kaplan had a double load of patients, his own and some of his partner's, but he took his time questioning me at length about my health history and Dr. Schultz's diagnosis of the current problem. In the examining room he ran the instrument that felt like razor blades over various areas of my feet and legs, stuck needles into the muscles and nerves, compared the feet for sensitivity, and bent, lifted, and pressed against my feet and legs to test muscle strength, control, and flexibility. He studied my bad gait.

After the examination, we returned to Dr. Kaplan's office. He began to talk to me while he dictated into his recorder. "I believe this lady does have spinal stenosis. I do not believe she should wait five weeks to do anything about it, however, in view of the speed at which the condition is worsening."

I seemed to feel the deterioration by the hour and it was my understanding that if a nerve remains cut off for very long and is damaged badly, it never regenerates completely. How many chances, I wondered, does a person get? How many times can I make a comeback?

While I listened, Dr. Kaplan phoned Dr. Schultz, who was almost out the door on his way to Africa, and discussed his diagnosis. Then he turned to me. "Dr. Schultz agrees with me that we should not wait to do something about your compressed nerve. He and I both believe you should go ahead and have a nerve root decompression as soon as the hospital can schedule it and, when Dr. Schultz gets back from his trip, he can do the anterior spinal fusion."

Oh, for some way out of this! There was silence as I considered all the implications an early surgery would have for the store. "Would you go ahead and schedule it?" I finally asked, my soul sinking.

"My nurse will make the appointment right now. Also, tomorrow I want you to go to the lab at Anna Kaseman Hospital for a blood-sugar test. I just want to be sure there aren't any interferences like diabetes."

That didn't bother me. My uncle Edwin had recently died of diabetes-related illnesses and I had hypoglycemia, but I knew I didn't have diabetes.

The nurse gave me a card with the appointment for surgery and she also instructed me about the blood-sugar test. "Go to the lab at eight tomorrow morning before you eat anything to have some blood drawn. Then go eat a regular breakfast and return at the end of two hours. They'll draw another syringe of blood and compare the levels of sugar in your blood at the two different times."

Limping and depressed, I left the medical building. Now I had only ten days, not twenty-seven, in which to do all the things that had to be done before I left the store. I'd be in the hospital about four weeks, not two. My orthopedic surgeon was out of the country, the neurosurgeon had never seen me before, and I had just changed to a new endocrinologist who hadn't even had a chance to get to know my particular system yet. He had completed his initial study of my health conditions and said, "You're not the ordinary, straight-off-the-rack patient, you know."

How could my timing be so bad?

Life, how can you be so perverse?

Chapter 9

PRAYERS
BY FIBER-OPTIC CABLE

The letters regarding closing the store went to all of the local businesses and banks we patronized in addition to the ones across the country, and the word spread rapidly to our customers. Rumors came back to us that I was dying of cancer, and the number of sympathetic people who phoned and came to the store to express their sorrow grew by the day. Everyone was kind enough to say, and mean it, that our store had made a mark on the town and they'd miss it.

Our staff assured people that I didn't have cancer, just a back problem, but that I needed to get it taken care of and that's why I would not be in the store much longer. As word spread that my back was the problem, a powerful series of episodes began to take place.

Pete Daskalos, a handsome young Greek millionaire and president of the board of the St. George Greek Orthodox Church, came to see me and said, "You're going to be all right, Lucy. I'm praying for you."

Shiraz Kassam, a tall, dusky, successful businessman and Mukhi of the Moslem Mosque, expressed his deepest regrets and said, "I'm praying for you every day."

Henry Tafoya, a sportscaster for a CBS affiliate, a very

religious Catholic, told me, "I'll light a candle for you and pray every day."

The Jewish president of a New York manufacturing company phoned. "God is taking care of you. I'll pray for your quick recovery."

Frederick Myers, an ordained minister with St. Aidan's Episcopalian Church, himself plagued with a health condition but always cheerful and optimistic, said, "You're in all our prayers. We hope you're up and going again right away."

Dee Foster, active in the Unitarian church, came to tell me, "I'm keeping you in my prayers."

Austin Dillon, a minister at the First United Methodist Church, said, "The Men's Prayer Group meets every morning for breakfast and we're praying for you."

June Michaels, recognized for her activities in Jewish affairs in Los Angeles and Jerusalem, phoned from Los Angeles. "You're in all my prayers and you're going to be just fine."

One couple, customers of ours, were faith healers. They came to see me at the store during the middle of a business day and, unabashed by curious glances from nearby shoppers, laid their hands on my lower back and hip, bowed their heads, and prayed for God to heal the broken fusion and take away the pain.

Never in my life had I experienced so much demonstrated love and concern and prayers that were offered from different religions and ethnic backgrounds but directed to a single Supreme Power. I was in awe. I felt as though all those messages were being translated into a single language, a language called "Godspeak," and relayed by an enormous fiber-optic cable to a God who couldn't possibly ignore that many people focused on one single purpose. He simply had to be attentive to that many supplications.

The time for checking into St. Joseph Hospital was from two to four o'clock in the afternoon. I stayed at the store until noon, finishing as many details as possible before turning the store over to Tom to manage. As I made my final rounds of the departments and told the staff good-bye, one of them said, "Now don't go out in public [meaning the hospital] wearing nightgowns from any other store."

As a good retailing season would have it, our lingerie department was sold out of the short gowns I'd need for the first few days after each operation. Later on I'd wear long gowns, sleepshirts, or pj's and I did have enough of them. Hoping that I wouldn't be recognized in somebody else's lingerie department, I went to Mervyn's and bought a couple of shorties.

From Mervyn's I drove directly to the hospital, checked in, and was taken to the eighth-floor Neurological Unit to get settled in.

The intake nurse came into my new room with a smile. "You're Lucy Dobkins. How are you?"

"I'm fine except that my life is in shreds," I answered sharply.

"Well!" the nurse exclaimed. "Let's talk about this." She put aside the patient intake forms and questionnaires and sat down beside Bed 1026-II.

Virginia Hanratty, the nurse, slender from playing tennis and carefully groomed, would endear herself to me for always being so perceptive, intelligent, good-humored, and calm during any of the emergencies in the Neurological Unit.

As she studied me she extinguished her easy smile and the sparkle in her eyes. She focused totally on my crooked posture, fatigued body, the pain lines in my face, and the tears welling in my eyes. "You're scheduled for a nerve root decompression tomorrow morning. Is that why you feel your life is in shreds?" she asked kindly.

"That's only part of it. For one thing, I have a new business that I have to sell because of my back. For another, I just finished building a new two-story town house and now I can hardly climb the stairs in it. Also, my mother is eighty-six years old and depends on me to do a lot of things for her: accounting and banking, business correspondence and insurance, shopping and errands, and medical appointments. I won't be able to do anything for her for a while and I don't know what she'll do without help. And," I hesitated, thinking I probably shouldn't say this to anyone, "how can I keep the romance of a lifetime alive and healthy if I'm always in and out of the hospital?" I clenched my jaws, trying to hold back tears of discouragement and pain, the constant, deep, wearing pain.

Without discussing my concerns, Virginia confidently wished me well with the surgery and picked up her questionnaires.

She surreptitiously blotted teardrops from her eyes and directed my attention to the questions.

"Do you know your height and weight?"

"I'm five-five and I weigh a hundred thirty-five pounds."

"Are you being treated for any health conditions?"

"Yes. Adrenal insufficiency. Hypothyroidism. Hypopituitarism. Hypogonadism. Degenerative osteoarthritis. Hiatus hernia. Sympathetic dystrophy. Gout. Polysistemic Candidiasis Albicans," I answered as she filled in the blanks on her forms.

"Are you taking any medications?"

"Yes, here's the list I carry when I travel. I take Cortisone Acetate®, Levothroid®, Spironolactone®, Maxide®, Ecotrin®, Tavist-1®, Zantac®, Sulfinpyrazone®, Allopurinol®, Nystatin®, and Depo-Estradiol®. I also take nonprescription magnesium gluconate, manganese, potassium, and most of the vitamins and minerals."

Virginia scanned the list showing the medications, dosages, and times. "Do you have any allergies?"

"Yes, I do," I said bitterly. "Painkillers, anti-inflammatories, antibiotics, and adhesive tape. Everything I'll need the most for the next few weeks."

I handed her another travel list, the one that showed thirty-six commonly prescribed medications that caused bad allergic reactions for me. My doctor had charted each reaction one by one and discontinued all of the prescriptions.

"Have you had any previous operations?" Virginia continued, not visibly reacting to my bitterness.

I hated intake interviews! They always made me feel like some kind of attention-seeking hypochondriac.

Virginia waited.

"Well, there was a spinal fusion of the cervical vertebrae 3-4 in August of 1976; a fusion of lumbar 4-5 in February 1983; lumbar 5-6 in December 1983; and lumbar 6 with sacro 1, also in December 1983. I had a nerve root decompression of lumbar 5-6 in February 1984. Twice, I've had operations to remove Orthofuse implants from my back. Also, I've had an appendectomy, a tonsillectomy, removal of the Fallopian tubes, and about eight operations for an injury to my leg."

Still not at all resigned to accepting any more surgery, I said angrily with a husky voice and a lump in my throat, "I don't want any more operations!"

Virginia put down her pen, looked directly into my eyes, matter-of-factly responded, "You want to walk, don't you?" and left the room.

What could I say?

It was my intention that while I was in the hospital this time none of my friends would have to do as much to help me as they had in the past. I didn't want them to feel as though they needed to launder any gowns or bring fresh supplies from home, so I packed enough gowns and cover-ups, pj's, sleepshirts, panties, and bras to last as long as I'd be in the hospital. There was a problem, though, when I tried to hang them in the little wardrobe in my room. The wardrobe was too short and too narrow for my things to fit.

Darlene, the nurse who was helping me unpack and put everything away, saw the problem, said, "I've got an idea," and left the room. She returned in a few minutes, wheeling in one of the racks they hang IV bottles from. She efficiently transferred the clothing to the IV rack and it was perfect! The gowns and cover-ups cleared the floor, I could easily see what was there and reach what I needed, and the rack could be rolled from room to room each time I was moved.

With a store full of designer lingerie, that's what I privately owned, of course, and that's what I brought to wear. Over the weeks it turned out to be a happy diversion to have the stuff hanging on the IV rack. Nurses, lab technicians, therapists, and doctors were always looking at the nightwear and I guess dreaming their own private fantasies. I almost wished I'd brought some of the cute and sexy nighties or the satin and lace gowns encrusted with pearls and rhinestones, the satin robes with marabou cuffs, or the silk teddies our models showed so beautifully with our mink coats at the country-club fashion shows. The elegant clothing was what I really liked.

As it was, the nurses teased me about the lingerie and Dr. Kaplan cracked, "What is this? The Lucy's Pillowtalk Annex?" If I were going to have to take that much teasing, I should have brought some of the high-heeled satin and marabou slippers, too. Instead I brought plain flat scuffs that I could slip my feet into without bending over, but Nurse Sally Lash pestered me from the first day to the last about them. "They don't give you any support. You need a slipper that holds your foot better. Ask one of your friends to go get you some. If they don't go, I'm going to get them myself!" Patty, her sister, and I had grown up together in the same church youth group so we went back a long way. With her naturally platinum hair, irrepressible sunniness, and expert care, she could badger me all she wanted to and get away with it.

I'd been in hospitals enough to know that I needed a few of my own things around me, things that gave me comfort at a time of discomfort. I planned carefully and brought some of my favorite things: the baby-size pillow with the blue satin cases, exactly the right size and softness to feel nice against the side of my face; a compartmentalized cosmetic tray that I could use to organize my hand cream, lotion, makeup, toothbrush and toothpaste, comb, brush, pen, pencil, and notepad so they'd be at my fingertips.

Remembering how long the nights in a hospital can be, I brought my favorite cocoa mug and some packets of hot chocolate and powdered spiced cider, knowing that if I asked, the nurses would fill my cup with hot water during the small hours of the night. I couldn't leave home without some peanut butter and pickles for late-night snacks, so I packed little jars of them and Stanford said he'd keep me supplied with fresh sandwich bread. I also took a little bottle of avocado oil and lemon juice, my favorite salad dressing. Finally, and probably the most important, were the supply of paperback books, cassette player, and collection of music.

Most of those things were fairly routine to take to the hospital. Not so routine were all the supplies I brought in order to keep our business running smoothly until it was sold: the ledgers, financial records, office supplies, calculator, Rolodex of names and numbers, personnel files, and work schedules. I asked for a private room with two beds: one bed to sleep in and the other for my office. I must have thought I was going to take a working vacation.

After previous back operations, I was tired, nervous, and

weepy, and I got along best in a quiet room where I was in control of the TV and radio, the number of visitors, and the doctors, nurses, and other medical people coming in and out. I just wanted silence and rest during those times. This time I intended to bounce back faster and carry on with my life, but I still wanted a quiet room.

Nurses came and went, took my vital signs, gave instructions, and changed me into a hospital gown. The nursing supervisor and nurses who had taken care of me in the past dropped in to welcome me back and they expressed their hopes that the nerve root decompression tomorrow would be easier than the other back operations were. The one question everyone asked was, "What went wrong and why did you have to come back?" They promised me they'd keep coming to see me even though they weren't on my case.

Colorful fresh flowers, humorous cards, and stuffed animals were arriving. My belongings were neatly put away and I was as ready emotionally as I'd ever be, but that wasn't very much.

Chapter 10

PLEASE, GOD,
LET IT BE IN TIME

Early in the evening Dr. Randy Maydew, the anesthesiologist for the surgery, came to talk with me about the schedule for that night and the following morning. "A nurse will be here in a few minutes to begin preparing you for surgery. She'll use an antiseptic to scrub your lower back, the area where the incision will be made, for ten minutes. Later in the evening she'll give you a mild sedative to help you relax during the night."

This is just another refresher course, I thought. My back's been scrubbed so many times it's a wonder there's any skin left.

"You won't be allowed anything to eat or drink after midnight," the doctor continued. "About 5:30 tomorrow morning you'll be awakened for your shower and then you'll receive another ten-minute back scrub. We'll give you a mild tranquilizer at about the same time to make you sleepy and the nurse will insert a catheter into your bladder and an IV needle into your wrist. About an hour later a medical attendant will bring a gurney to your room and take you to the holding area for the operating room."

This was the same old song and not any sweeter.

"Your surgeon will be there to do your nerve root decompression and I will be there to give you the anesthetic. I'll stay with you every minute of the operation to monitor your vital signs and make any necessary adjustments in the solution you'll be receiving."

I didn't need to ask what was next. This was Operation No. 19 in my life and the doctor's next line was going to be "After the operation . . ."

Dr. Maydew, puzzled by the look of cynicism on my face, continued. "After the operation, we'll take you to the recovery room until we're certain you're coming out of the anesthesia without any problems and then we'll bring you back to this floor and place you in the Advanced Neurological Unit, Intensive Care, where you'll have a nurse with you continuously to monitor your recovery. Your doctor will determine when you're ready to return to your own room."

The anesthesiologist, a good-looking, likable young man, asked about my health history, present health conditions, and any medications I was taking on a regular basis. I gave him my travel list. Dr. Maydew took the list and studied it carefully. "I'm concerned about the number of health conditions you have and the medications you need. I'm especially concerned, though, about the number of drugs you're allergic to. Who is your endocrinologist?"

"Dr. William Mitchell. He said he'd be coming here at about this time this evening."

The anesthesiologist said, "I'll need to consult with him tonight before I can plan your anesthetic. Do you have any questions before I go?"

"No, none. Thanks for talking to me."

The doctor left as my night nurse came in to begin the pre-op activities. "You'll need to remove your nail polish so the true color of your fingernails can be watched. It helps the doctors know about your circulation. You'll probably hate me for this, but you'll have to give up your artificial eyelashes. If an eyelid were to roll inward while you were lying on your face during surgery, the artificial lashes could cause damage to your eye," she said as she began the scrub.

Short, wrinkled, cotton hospital gown. No nail polish. No makeup. No eyelashes. No contact lenses. I was becoming a basic starter kit, I thought with disgust.

At ten o'clock the nurse brought my regular medications and

a sleeping pill. Before I became drowsy I looked over the personal belongings I'd brought for taking care of myself and was satisfied that they were organized in such a way as to be the most convenient and useful to me.

I took a late-night walk in the halls just to keep using my muscles for as long as possible, acutely aware of the cold numbness in my foot, the heavy, constant pain in my lower leg, the deteriorating ankle strength, and the never-ending ache in my back and hip.

Slipping into bed and pulling up the covers, I said a simple, silent prayer. "Please, God, let this nerve root decompression be successful. Let it be in time to keep me from becoming crippled again."

The nurse, energetic and cheery even at the end of her long day, came in to wish me luck for tomorrow and to pull up the side rails on the bed.

During the endless night I slept fitfully, awakening often to the sounds of the nurses talking to patients as they went from room to room. "How are you feeling? I'm going to take your temperature, okay?" Occasionally I could hear the plop and scrape of a walker as a sleepless patient shuffled slowly down the corridor. Metal doors to the fire stairs opened and banged shut as lab technicians took the short route down to their laboratory. The wheels on the medication cart squealed as the cart was pushed from room to room. Telephones rang. An all-night TV show played in some room nearby. Toilets flushed.

There were shouts of pain and pleas for a nurse to please come quickly. I could hear soft moans and sobs and I couldn't really separate which ones were someone else's and which ones were my own.

The surgery was finished.

At some time during the night I began to awaken enough to realize that this was probably the Advanced Neurological Unit, Intensive Care.

Stanford had come to the hospital every hour throughout the day to check on me and he'd finally remained until I was awake enough to talk to him. Bea, Barnett, and Wess had been at the hospital all day, too, waiting for reports from the doctor and a chance to see for themselves that I was fine.

As I became fully conscious, the enormity of the pain in my back was too overwhelming to endure. In a hoarse whisper, the best sound I could make with my dry throat, I called to the nurse. "This hurts so much! Can you give me something to stop the pain, please?"

The nurse read the orders in my chart, brought a pill, and held a straw in a glass of water for me to sip and swallow. As minutes passed and became an eternity, there was no relief from the pain.

"That pill didn't help at all. Can't you give me something that will work?" I croaked, my throat dry and sore from tubes and anesthetic.

The nurse in Intensive Care had worked there for many years—someone had already reassured me that I'd have good care—so I was sure she probably knew her business: to do what was best for her patients. But in my tortured, semilucid state, I saw her only as cold and uncaring when she said, "That's the only painkiller your doctor ordered."

It seemed as though hours passed. The pain was full blown and wild and I begged, now humbled by the agony, for something that would help.

"All right!" the nurse retorted with a short temper. "I'll call your doctor and see what he says!" When she returned she said, "Your neurosurgeon has ordered another painkiller for you to take. Swallow this."

"What kind is it?" I questioned before I swallowed it. My question came out sounding as though I was ungrateful, but all I meant was that I wanted to be sure it was a drug that wouldn't cause me a problem. I didn't want any more problems of any kind. I couldn't handle what I had already.

She told me the name and I exploded. "I can't take that! I'm allergic to it. It's in all my records, right on the front with a red label. Why'd you give me that? Call the doctor back and get something I can take!"

The nurse said sternly, "I've already made one call in the night to your doctor at home and that's all the calls you get!"

Oh, God! What can I do? This agony is more than I can stand but if I take that pill, I'll turn into a total itch from my head to my feet. It'll make me crazy!

The nurse stood waiting, the pill in her hand. Some choice! "I'll take the pill," I said grimly and sipped enough water through the straw to swallow it.

Twenty minutes later, going wild with itching, I asked again for help.

"Now what's going on?" the nurse demanded.

"I'm reacting to the painkiller. I itch everywhere—in my hair and eyes, face and ears, and all over my body. Do you have something to stop it?"

The nurse looked at my purplish coloring and watched my frantic scratching, then called another nurse to stay with me while she went to get a syringe of Benadryl®. She gave me the injection and the itching quickly subsided. I sank, exhausted, into a blinding fog of pain and half-sleep.

Every two hours a team of nurses came in and awakened me, firmly grasped the edges of the drawsheet, and turned my body to a different position. "You can't stay on your back any longer than this. It's not good for you. We know you're miserable and we're trying to be gentle, but we do have to turn you."

Tears slipped from under my closed lids and down my face and when they left I tried to squirm into any tiny change of position that would be something I could stand.

At the end of an endless night, Dr. Kaplan made his morning rounds and came to stand beside my bed. "There was more of a problem than I expected when I got in where I could look at your spine. You had two levels, not just one, where the nerves from the spine were blocked. I cleaned out a lot of fragments of debris and I scraped the bony overgrowth away from the spinal openings in order to free the nerves. The areas are clean now, the nerves are free, and you're going to be just fine." He studied my chart, wrote new orders for my medications, and then directed the nurses to transfer me out of the Advanced Neurological Unit into my own room. "I want you to gain strength as fast as you can in order to be ready for the spinal fusion in two weeks," he said. "I'm ordering a particularly nutritious diet with supplemental fluids, daytime rest, and something to help you sleep soundly at night. I want you to have as much physical exercise as you can tolerate as quickly as possible, so I'll have the physical therapists come in to work with you and get you on your feet and walking."

He wished me a good day and assured me the nurses would call him if I had any problems.

Chapter 11

MAYBE A PSYCHOLOGIST CAN HELP

Dear God,

I talk to you a lot. All the time, in fact. I don't think I'm
ever rude or unreasonable or demanding, but now I'm
mad and it's you I'm made at! How could you let this happen? I went through all of this three years ago. You were
there. You saw it all. You know how hard it was. Where are
you anyway?

My first impression that Dr. Kaplan was cool and distant and
that he was only taking care of me in order to help his sick partner changed very quickly. Dr. Kaplan came to see me every
morning, always earlier than any of the other doctors. He
watched attentively as I tried unsuccessfully to move my foot up,
down, or from side to side, and when he told me to exert pressure with my foot against his hand, my foot wouldn't move. It
was also still icy cold.

I was certain the operation was a failure. My foot was as bad as
it was before and now my back was even worse. Yet Dr. Kaplan
kept assuring me, "Your foot is going to be fine. The nerves are
bruised and swollen now, but as the swelling goes down, you'll
begin to get back the use of your foot. I want you to try to exercise it throughout the day, every day. Keep trying to move it up
and down and from side to side."

Darlene Williams, the nurse accompanying Dr. Kaplan on his rounds, said, "Dr. Kaplan's right. You can trust him. You're going to be fine. I'll come back in a little while to help you with your exercises and get you bathed and dressed." Darlene's duty day began each morning at seven and she was one of the most important nurses in my recovery.

A few days after the surgery, as Dr. Kaplan finished asking me questions and examining my foot and the incision in my back, he looked at me intently, a serious expression on his face, and said, "I'd like to have Reid Hester see you. Dr. Hester is a psychologist with a special interest in patients who have long-term chronic pain and the problems of rehabilitation. I think you're going through some pretty hard times right now. Maybe a psychologist can help."

A psychologist? That was a surprise! I hadn't pegged Dr. Kaplan as being able to see into my head at all. Equally surprising, and I took it personally and felt demeaned, was the suggestion that I, a counselor with a certain amount of recognition of my own, move to the other side of the desk and be the one counseled. That hit hard at my pride in being able to solve my own problems.

Do I look sick? That sick? I questioned myself. Is this how my own clients feel when I suggest that they see a psychologist? What will my friends and family say if I tell them I'm going to see a psychologist?

Well, if I'm going to be honest with myself, I have to admit that yes, I am sick, and bravado isn't going to do me any good this time. I'm not going to be able to pull myself out of this one without some help so I'd better take it when it's offered.

I consented.

"Good. This psychologist can help you. I'll talk with him today and ask him to drop around to see you."

The psychologist, tall, suntanned from sailing in Australia, and good-looking, reminding me of my brother, came striding into the room the next morning. He introduced himself and sat down beside the bed. "Dr. Kaplan told me that a lot of things have happened to you in a short period of time and that you're having a bit of a hard time coping with them."

Filled with pain and discouragement, unable to use my foot,

uncertain of what my future was, I had to acknowledge that yes, this certainly was a hard time. I said with bile in my voice, "The way I look at life is that God watches all of us in about the same interested way that we watch the characters on TV dramas in their day-to-day lives. This time, though, when He saw 'The Days and Nights of Lucy Dobkins' coming on again, He went out for popcorn and I don't know if He's ever coming back!" I broke down and cried.

Dr. Hester quietly waited until I could compose myself and then said, "I'd like for you to fill out three tests which will help me reach an early understanding of how you're feeling about some important areas in your life. I'd like for you to allow me to try to help you work through the areas that are troubling you."

He handed me some test folders and said, "This test is the Minnesota Multiphasic Personality Inventory. It consists of 566 true and false questions. The Millon Behavior Health Inventory has 150 true and false questions and the Beck Inventory has 21 forced-choice statements. It'll take you part of the afternoon to fill out the tests and I can pick them up at the end of the day and have them scored by computer overnight. I can talk with you about the results tomorrow morning. Is that all right with you?"

I nodded.

"Do you have any questions?"

I didn't. Those tests were some that I gave my own clients. I already knew what they were for.

Dr. Hester left the tests with me and said, "Good. I'll see you later this evening," and left.

I'd always tried to be understanding of my clients' apprehension about being examined in this way, but this experience made me even more empathetic.

Now that I was the one being examined, I wondered how reliable the tests really were and how bad I was going to look on them.

Dr. Hester came back with the test results the next morning.

Frightened to ask, but compelled to know, I asked, "How did I look on the tests?"

Dr. Hester was entirely straightforward. "Your Beck score

indicated that you are significantly clinically depressed and borderline suicidal."

Dead silence.

My heart sank and my face felt a rush of heat from the embarrassment that the test was revealing my true state of mind, which, up to now, was secret to anyone except me.

"That is corroborated by the MMPI. Also, the evaluation instruments indicate a significant need for self-control and self-mastery and that tells me that it will be important that your doctors and nurses increase your involvement in managing your medications and physical therapy. The Millon shows you have a calm demeanor which gets significantly ruffled at the demands of others, social criticism, or severe illness."

Although I carefully had not revealed my feelings of hopelessness to anyone, I knew the test results were all true and that I did need help to get well physically and emotionally. I wasn't in control of my life anymore and I didn't know how to get control. "What I want is to get well and get my normal way of life back. What do I have to do?" I asked tiredly.

"Your doctors want to do several things," Dr. Hester said. "First, they don't want you to be taking any pain medication at all by the time you go into surgery ten days from now. They want nature and your body to take over more of the control of pain before your body has to rely on some temporary assistance from pain medications. They want you to begin physical therapy to build up as much muscle strength as you can before the spinal fusion is performed. And I'd like to see you for an hour a day."

"How long do you think you'll need to see me?" I asked.

"You're strong, you're resilient, and you're willing to work toward getting well. I think I'll need to see you for four to six months," Dr. Hester answered. "You'll need to work on accepting the fact that you'll probably live at a high level of pain for the rest of your life, but there are ways of handling it to make it less of an interference in your daily life. We're going to work on those ways. Such things as distraction, physical and mental, will help keep you from dwelling on your pain. Breaking up your activities into smaller time blocks and resting in between will put less strain on your body. Completely avoiding those physical activities which are damaging to backs will be essential. There are relaxation techniques you can learn to relieve tension that worsens back problems. Equally necessary will be the reduction of stress in your life. Your doctor told me how many hours you were working in your store because you wanted it to be a success. It wasn't smart before this operation and it'll be damn stupid to even think about it from now on. You'll have to learn some entirely different kind of work from any of the careers you've had before. What that will be I don't know, but we're going to explore it together. I know you're resentful at having to give up for the second time a profession you loved, and I understand, but we're going to deal with that too."

Dr. Hester hesitated and waited for my reaction. I remained silent.

"We'll also explore the reasons you seem compelled to act like Superwoman and do a million things and try to do all of them perfectly. I'll work with you on ways to moderate that way of life."

That touched a nerve! Offended now, I objected. "It's hard for me to change the way I act! Almost everybody in my family acts that way, all my friends act that way, and my nine-year-old granddaughter is seeing a child psychologist because she acts ·that way too. It just looks normal to me."

"I know. During the months ahead, we're going to unravel those problem areas in your life and reweave them into new attitudes and behaviors that will be healthier for you," Dr. Hester responded.

I consented to have the therapy.

"Good!" Dr. Hester said. "The first thing I'd like for you to do is ask one of your friends to pick up two books that have information and suggestions that I think will be helpful to you. One is a book called *Feeling Good,* by David Burns, M.D., and the other one is *Managing Chronic Pain: A Patient's Guide,* by C. David Tollison, Ph.D."

As he left, Bea and Barnett came in. I told them who Dr. Hester was and explained what was happening. Bea, formerly in social work, and Barnett, who had been a parole officer working with prisoners and their families, understood the value of therapy and both of them supported me in my decision.

I gave them the names of the books Dr. Hester

recommended, but said, "Bea, you are still getting over your open-heart surgery and I don't want to tax you in any way. If you happen to be in a bookstore, it would be nice if you'd buy these two books for me, but don't make any special trips to do it."

"We'll stop at the bookstore on our way home and bring them to you tomorrow," she answered. "We spend all our time in bookstores anyway, so this isn't a special trip." They kissed my cheek and left.

Everyone gone, I lay alone with my thoughts. So I'm to have therapy! Instead of me talking with people, winning their trust and drawing out their deepest thoughts and emotions, I'm now expected to trust someone else, a stranger, bare my very private soul, throw away the coping mechanisms I've learned from a lifetime of experiences and start my life all over again. It's an impossible task! I'm not rigid and set in my ways, but I'm not jelly either. And I'm tired!

Maybe I can't succeed and maybe I can't change my way of life.

Maybe I'm just so depressed I don't even care.

Chapter 12

ONE DOWN
AND ONE TO GO

Between the operations, with all the reports on radio and television and in newspapers and magazines, I became concerned about the risk of catching serious diseases from blood transfusions. I hadn't needed any transfusions during the nerve root decompressions and, when I asked Dr. Kaplan about spinal fusions, he said there usually wasn't any need for blood transfusions during that kind of surgery either. He did think it was a good idea, however, for me to donate blood for myself and have it held in reserve just in case, since my blood type wasn't the most common one and supplies in the blood bank were often limited. Dr. Kaplan suggested that I self-donate only as much blood as would be safe for me to give between two major operations so close together. He said he'd arrange for a United Blood Services nurse to come talk with me.

The lady who came to see me was a friendly, cute, efficient nurse who had retired from hospital nursing and now worked as a volunteer for the bank. She answered all of my questions and assured me that my own blood, if I self-donated, would be labeled and held completely separate from any other blood. "I can draw one unit, a pint, today and another one tomorrow if that's what you decide you want to do, but that's all the doctor will allow you to give this close to a second surgery. There's an adequate supply of your Type A Negative blood in the blood bank now, however, and it's safe blood. We'll have some from the bank tagged and ready on the shelves in the operating room when you go in for your surgery and, if it turns out that you do need a blood transfusion and your own two pints aren't enough, it will all be ready."

Wanting to know where the bank gets its blood, I asked the volunteer, "What are your requirements for donors?"

"We require that a donor be over seventeen years of age and weigh a minimum of 110 pounds. We don't accept blood from anyone who's had hepatitis, cancer within the last ten years, diabetes requiring insulin, or anyone who used drugs intravenously or had exposure to an individual or a group at high risk of contracting AIDS. All of our blood donations must pass certain screening tests to make sure they are free from contamination."

"I do want to donate to myself. When can you do it?" I asked.

"Right now," she answered and prepared her equipment: a tourniquet on my arm, a needle, and a tube to carry the blood to a container.

It was easy to donate. I just lay there.

The nurse finished, put away her equipment, and said, "Your nurse will bring you some grape juice to drink and I want you to drink plenty of other fluids, too. You might be a little weak or dizzy now, so stay in bed for the rest of the day. You mustn't take any chances of falling. Tomorrow I'll come back and draw the other unit of blood." The volunteer nurse left, carrying her little container.

Still apprehensive about using any public blood despite the assurance of protective measures, I told Stanford and Wess that evening about the conversation with the nurse. "I've already donated one pint of blood for myself and I'll donate another pint tomorrow."

Both of them said they wanted to be my donors and they volunteered to sit next to the operating room all during the next operation in case they were needed for blood. As it turned out, though, we had different blood types and our blood wasn't compatible; just our personalities were!

I rather liked the idea of Stanford's blood being transfused into mine. "It reminds me of being a little kid," I laughed, "when my best friend and I nicked our skin and stirred our blood together so that we'd become blood sisters."

"If you and I mixed our blood, would that make our relationship incestuous?" Stanford joked.

"Oh . . . bad!" I groaned and turned both thumbs down.

When Bea and Barnett came to visit, we talked about the news reports of AIDS and how it was spread from one person to another. They said, "We've just heard about a fine hotel in Glasgow where the maids ordinarily go through all of the rooms each night, turn down the sheets, and place a chocolate mint on each pillow. The hotel has recently changed its policy, though, and now when the maids turn down the sheets they place a condom instead of a mint on each pillow." Bea, in her late seventies, and Barnett, in his eighties, married to each other for fifty-four years and looking forward to their next vacation trip, said with enthusiasm, "We don't want the condoms. We want the chocolate mints!"

The operations were one down and one to go. During the sixteen days between them the nurses helped me sit up on the side of the bed and dangle my feet. That was a Big Ow-ee! In a few days I could stand up and my back bore the weight of my body, but it made plenty of objections. By the end of the week I could, with the nurses' help, transfer from the side of the bed to the bedside commode, but I couldn't decide which was worse: trying to arch my back enough while lying in bed to have a bedpan placed under my bottom, or having to sit up, stand up, then sit down on this low commode, and then having to reverse the maneuver to get back into bed.

The physical therapists came each day, buckled the heavy webbed belt around my waist for them to hold on to to keep me from falling, and helped me use a walker to begin taking steps. Within a few more days, with their help, I could support myself with the walker well enough to walk from the side of the bed across the room to the doorway to the hall.

"Our next goal for you," the therapists said at the end of a session, "is for you to increase your strength and prepare for the next operation. We also want you to become able to climb your stairs when you go home. Starting tomorrow we're going to take you down the hall to the fire stairs and assist you until you can climb all twelve steps, turn around safely at the top, and walk back down. You're going to learn to step up with your good foot and step down with your bad one. That's going to be your mantra: up with the good one, down with the bad one."

I was making healthy gains and showing it. Everybody was pleased.

Control of the pain was still a major problem and Bea and Barnett suffered over it as much as I did. One afternoon they came in with a suggestion. "We were telling our daughter in Chicago, Ruthie, about your allergies to pain medication and she said she'd been at a party with some doctors from Northwestern University Hospital who were talking about a patient from Canada that they had fitted with an electronic pain device called a TENS Unit. Ruthie was able to obtain the patient's phone number but not her name. She thinks you should phone her in Canada and find out all you can."

They handed me the phone number. I dialed it and when a woman answered I introduced myself, told her how I happened to have her telephone number, and said, "I'm in the hospital for back surgery and I'm allergic to painkillers. Would you mind telling me about the electronic device you're using?"

The Canadian volunteered her name and address so that I could reach her by letter in addition to telephone and said, "I'd love to! This device has changed my life! I have a bad back that's had several operations but it still isn't good and there isn't anything more that can be done for it. The pain was ruining my life and my marriage. I couldn't cook, couldn't clean house, couldn't work, and couldn't do things for my husband or children. Since I got the TENS I'm able to cook and keep house, I do my own grocery shopping, my disposition has improved, and so have my relations with my family."

She told me all the details of her back problems and what kind of device the TENS was. "I think you should ask your doctor about getting one for you. If he doesn't have one, he'll know where he can get it." She wished me as much success as she was having and we said good-bye.

What strange and unexpected things can happen through a chain of friends!

I talked with Dr. Kaplan about the TENS. He did know about

it and wrote an order for the Physical Therapy Department to provide one for me and show me how to use it.

The physical therapists brought a unit the next morning and explained it. "TENS, for Transcutaneous Electronic Nerve Stimulation, is an electronic unit designed on the principle that the electrical currents it transmits act to produce a release of the brain's own opiates and therefore relieve pain. We'll clip this small battery case to your gown." The therapists demonstrated. "We'll plug the ends of the wires into the battery unit and the other ends into these small patches with this gel which conducts current and then attach them to the areas of your body where the pain is the greatest, like this." They stuck the patches onto the two places that hurt the most in my lower back.

"These dials on the battery unit are what you control. This dial controls the rate of pulsation from the unit," a therapist said as she had me turn the control both directions and feel the change in pulsation. "This other dial regulates the strength of the stimulations. They'll feel a little bit like electric shocks, but they don't hurt unless you turn the intensity too high."

I tested it and found out what she meant. When the therapists were sure I understood how to operate the unit, they left it fitted to me, reminded me to be careful not to pull out the electric wires when I turned over or moved around, and gave me their phone number to call if I had any trouble with the unit before they came back tomorrow.

So this is a TENS! An electronic marvel! Was it really going to stop the pain, I wondered, or was it just going to be so much of a distraction with its wires and pulsations that I'd forget the pain? Either way was all right with me. I wanted to stop hurting and I didn't care how I did it.

This period between operations seemed like a good time to practice a technique for bringing about relaxation and a sense of well-being that a professor from California had presented to some of us at a seminar in Santa Fe. "This exercise," our instructor had begun in a soothing voice, "is to help you reach a state of relaxation which allows your body to release tension and free your energy to work towards higher levels of accomplishment and self-confidence, and greater degrees of physical well-being. You're going to create in your mind an image of how you want to be. This is what I want you to do."

We were in a college lounge that was carpeted and furnished with comfortable overstuffed couches and chairs. A fresh breeze off the Sangre de Cristo Mountains swept the fragrance of pine trees through the open windows. Our instructor seated herself in the middle of the floor, yoga style.

"I don't want you to talk to anyone until after we've finished. Don't move around the room or do anything that might distract someone else. Just find a place where you can sit or lie down comfortably." She had paused for everyone to get settled.

In a calm and quiet voice she began to talk again. "I want you to begin to breathe very slowly and deeply. Close your eyes. Begin relaxing all of your muscles, one at a time. Wrinkle up your forehead as high as you can and then drop it and feel the tension go out of it. Relax your eyelids. Think about how much you are relaxing. Relax your jaws and chin and the tension in the back of your neck and between your shoulder blades. Shrug your shoulders as hard as you can and then let them drop. Do it again. Let your shoulders drop in total, complete relaxation. Think about how relaxed you are. Move your thoughts to your arms and hands, your chest, stomach, and buttocks. Move the relaxed feelings down each leg and into your feet and toes. Pull your toes toward your chin, tighten your ankles as much as you can, and then release your toes to fall down relaxed. Think about how relaxed you are all over your body. You're perfectly calm and quiet. Keep breathing slowly, deeply, evenly."

In my hospital bed I followed the instructions as I remembered them.

"Now," my recollection said, "bring to your mind the image of a happy memory. Remember every detail of it: where you were, everything that belongs in the picture, the scenery, colors, smells, and sounds. Add to your picture any person who was with you and think of how that person looked and what you said to each other. Think about the feelings you were having during that happy moment. Lock that image in your mind so that you can flip a switch in your mind at any time and transport yourself back to that happy moment whenever you want to." The instructor stopped talking then and waited quietly for a few minutes.

"What you'll do next is project yourself into the future and create in your mind what time period it is, where you are, and why you're there. Now think about what you need to do or be in order to make the picture exactly what you want for yourself in real life, not just in your imagination. Do you want to be thinner? Create an image of yourself as thinner and study how you look and how your clothes fit. Do you want to be strong, healthy, and vital? Bring that image into focus. Do you want to be more productive, efficient, and organized? Paint the picture showing you being those things in the very setting where you want to display them. Hold on to your image for a little longer. Study it for every detail. Determine what you need to do in real life to look like the image in your mind."

Now, quietly, I created images of myself as slender, tan, and barefooted, hair blowing in the sea breeze as I swung along the ocean shore with white-tipped surf rolling toward the beach to cool my toes. There wasn't any limp in my gait or any stiffness in my back. In my image I easily bent down and picked up seashells washed ashore. I leaped skyward to catch a stray ball from the kids up the beach and tossed it back without a twinge of pain. That was how I wanted to be.

It did help for me to relax and to project myself into a better condition, but there was still the reality that I was in enormous pain and there wasn't much pain medication I could safely take. At the times when the hurting was so bad that I really couldn't stand it anymore, the nurses gave me an injection of the one intravenous medication that hadn't caused any problems for me. We were grateful for even one intravenous painkiller that we could still rely on.

When Darlene came on duty at seven one morning, I said to her, "It's been a really hard night. I'm hurting too much to go on any longer without something to stop it. Could you give me a shot, please?"

Darlene hurried out to get the medication and returned quickly. "This will make you feel better. I'll be back in a few minutes to set up your bath and freshen your bed."

When she returned, she looked at me unusually closely and asked, "Do you feel all right?"

"Yes, I feel a lot better now, thanks." Then, curious at the tone of her voice, I asked, "Why?"

"Because your face, neck, and chest are turning purple!" she exclaimed.

Within five minutes I was a madwoman, crazy from the terrible itching in my eyes and ears, face and hair, body, legs, and arms. There wasn't any place that didn't itch. Damn! Darlene raced to the nurses' station and returned with a syringe of Benadryl®. Within twenty minutes the itching calmed down and the purplish color began to leave my face. Thoughtfully regarding me, Darlene asked, "What do you suppose would happen if we gave you the Benadryl® first the next time, waited ten minutes, and then gave you the painkiller?"

"I don't know, but let's try it. Would you talk with the doctor?"

Dr. Kaplan agreed to let us try it and wrote the order. From then on that was the procedure the nurses used for all of my injections of pain medications. Mr. Benadryl®, I think I owe you a night on the town for all of this!

Now we only knew of one painkiller by pill and one that was given intravenously that I didn't react to and we all knew to expect considerable pain again when the next operation was done. In order to continue decreasing the amount of painkiller I was presently taking, the doctors changed the medication from shots and pills to pain cocktails.

"The pain cocktail," Dr. Hester explained to me, "has the same level of narcotic you're now taking but in liquid form. Pain cocktails will be given to you on a regular time schedule rather than on a pain-contingent basis. That way you won't reinforce the pain by rewarding it with a shot or a pill, and your body will be forced to adapt. Also we're going to systematically reduce the amount of narcotic as rapidly as you can tolerate the loss of it,"

"I'll be glad to try the pain cocktails," I said. "One of those painkillers causes me cold chills alternating with perspiration, and I'm nauseous a lot."

Weirdest of all, though, and I didn't tell him this, were the brilliant, spinning, psychedelic dreams the painkillers gave me. My entire "movie screen" of viewing was filled with gigantic male organs accompanied by huge orgasms—mine! It was a strange sensation and puzzling, especially since I had always thought I was such a nice girl.

In the meantime, Dr. Kaplan continued to check my foot and back every morning. He assured me, "The nerves in your foot are responding to pinpricks and the use of your foot is going to return. Keep trying all the time to move it up and down and from side to side. You're going to be fine. Your foot might always stay cold, though, and you'll just have to learn to live with it."

More and more frequently doctors were saying to me, "You're just going to have to live with it." Pretty soon I might as well not even try to get anything fixed. What difference was it going to make? my thoughts were asking. I'll just end up having to learn to live with it anyway.

My brothers and sister were phoning regularly from around the country, and my son in Denver brought his two little girls and a friend to see me several times. Business associates continued to call and write cards of encouragement and love. My room was a garden of beautiful flowers, which Wess volunteered to take care of every day, quietly tiptoeing around the room in her stockings.

I was beginning to feel relatively good and I enjoyed talking with everyone who came to see me. People always asked me, "How are you?" My answer varied like the value of the American dollar on the world currency market: one day it was a rising dollar, and the next day it was a falling dollar, but I was generally on the up side.

Dick Neal, my principal until he retired because of heart surgery, brought an American Beauty rose and vase for my night table and we reminisced and laughed about the fun we had when we worked together.

Peter Grivas, our interior designer for the store, kept me up-to-date on his projects in Albuquerque and Santa Fe and told me what various business associates of ours were doing. We talked about his years as an architect and interior designer in Mexico City and, more recently, his ministerial work with prison inmates. I was fascinated by the variety of his experiences.

Henry Tafoya, the sportscaster, dropped in to chat. In addition to reporting all the sports news for a CBS affiliate, he also owned a company that made commercial films. While I was still in the store, we had held some conversations about making a lingerie promotion film. Two of the major lingerie manufacturing companies had tested the market with the idea and it looked promising.

It was always stimulating, too, when Dolores ("Dody") Hoffman came to see me. Fifteen years ago, Dody, the Bittners, and I all moved to the same apartment complex when it first opened and we often met each other at the swimming pool on Saturday mornings when we squeezed an hour out of our schedules to swim. Dody, a division supervisor in purchasing at Sandia National Laboratories, was always commuting between Albuquerque; Oak Ridge, Tennessee; Livermore, California; the Nevada Test Site; and Washington, D.C. Dody is little and chic and so funny she made my stitches hurt. Her husband, Jim, is a handsome, low-key but high-voltage physicist doing sophisticated research for Sandia National Labs. When Dody isn't in Washington, Dr. Hoffman is.

I needed the lively conversations with my friends, and hearing what they were doing helped me begin to put my own life into a better perspective.

Stanford came to my room every morning at 6:30 and I always looked forward to seeing him. I tried to wake up early enough to freshen up, put on my makeup, and brush my hair before he got there. He brought yogurt with fruit, milk, and a Danish to share while we talked. We even took some morning walks, even if they were only a hundred steps with a walker. We wanted to keep our good life of early breakfasts, interesting conversations, and healthy walks, so we just made a few adaptations and went ahead with them.

We had a moment of laughter when Darlene came on shift ahead of schedule one morning and happened to walk in on breakfast with Stanford. "So that's why your blood pressure is never the same at this time of day as it is the rest of the time!" she laughed as she grinned meaningfully at Stanford and excused herself. Poor Stanford! He had endeared himself to the nurses with his good humor and constant care of me and they loved to embarrass him.

Physically and emotionally I was getting better. Dr. Hester spent an hour with me every morning, helping me identify the behaviors that were not in my own best interest. With his help I began to recognize that I am much too driven and, inevitably, it defeats me. He persuaded me that not everyone pushes himself to that extreme and that there's nothing wrong in taking a more relaxed approach to my work. We spent a lot of time working through my grief over giving up the store and, still making me unhappy, the loss of my counseling work. While I'd searched in my mind as many vocations and professions as I knew about and discarded them as not appropriate for me anymore, Dr. Hester took the approach of having me list the things I knew how to do that didn't require the best back in the world.

Our conversations were stormy, angry, tearful, and sad. I ran the gamut of emotions as I tried to pull out of the deep well of depression I was in.

As he got up to leave one morning, Dr. Hester said, "Your job for tomorrow is to think about all your many friends and pick one to have come here regularly for you to talk to her or him about all these worries that are eating away at you. Pick someone who will listen without judging, criticizing, or giving advice. I'll ask you tomorrow who it is."

All day and all night I thought about my friends from every aspect of friendship. There were so many and they were so good to me, how could I choose? This would be a heavy-duty job for anyone who accepted and I needed to be sure I didn't ask too much of any of them.

Dr. Hester asked as soon as he entered the room the next morning, "Did you choose a friend?"

"Yes, I did."

"Who is it?"

"I chose Dee Foster."

"Tell me about Dee Foster," he commanded.

"Dee is a small, reddish-blonde fireball with more talent and energy than you'd ever expect to find. She's extremely intelligent, very sensitive, a bit earthy, and lots of fun. If anyone threatens to do damage to someone she cares about, she's as gutsy as a mother lion with a den full of cubs. We used to work together when Dick Neal was our principal and Dee is part of the reason that our school had such a good curriculum and we all had so much fun. She works now in the school district's administrative office in a consulting and advising type of position for all of the language-arts teachers in the system. She presents workshops to update teaching techniques, helps with the selection of textbooks in the state, works with the legislature, and does so

many other things that I don't even know what they all are. I
do know I can trust her with my life. We've traded confidences
during each other's moments of crisis for a long time."
"Call her," Dr. Hester ordered. "Tell her I'd like to meet her
sometime when it's convenient for her. Now let's talk about the
pros and cons of you being a consultant to entrepreneurs and
retailers and teaching classes in how to start and run a business."

After Dr. Hester left, I telephoned Dee at her office. "Dee,
I've told you a little bit about Dr. Hester and now I need to ask
a big favor of you. He told me to choose a friend I could talk to
about anything that bothered me and just be my sounding
board, not judge and not give advice. I'd like for it to be you.
Can you come over anytime soon?"

"Of course! I'll be there at 4:30 today if that's all right with
you," Dee answered just as though she had all the time in the
world, which she didn't. She lived a fast pace and worked at a
demanding job and I knew she'd have to shuffle her schedule in
order to see me.

When she arrived I explained. "Dr. Hester said I have a lot
of uncertainties and worries that I need to talk about and work
through. Would it be possible to see you regularly until I can get
my head on straight?"

"Yes, it is and I'm glad you chose me. That's an honor. I can
be here every day. You just tell me what time is best for you so
that I don't come when you're resting or seeing your doctors
or physical therapists."

We arranged a schedule that suited both of us and began a
series of serious, often emotional, conversations that helped me
put everything into better perspective and be able to move
ahead with my life.

Chapter 13

ANTERIOR SPINAL FUSION

Dr. Schultz had scheduled an operating room for March 28 to do an anterior spinal fusion and that would be the day after tomorrow, but no one had heard from him. I was getting nervous. Then, during the middle of the sunny spring afternoon, he walked into my room fresh from the wild, exotic sights of Africa. He seemed glad to see me and I was certainly glad to see him!

"I called your home and no one answered, so I called your store to talk with you about your surgery. Your manager said you weren't there and when I asked where I could find you, he said I could find you lying in a bed at St. Joseph Hospital and said you'd been there for two weeks waiting for me to operate on you. I thought I better get down here and find out what's been going on," Dr. Schultz said with chagrin.

"Well, here I am, just waiting. Dr. Kaplan did the nerve root decompressions on March 11th and I've been here getting well ever since. Is everything set for the spinal fusion the day after tomorrow?" I asked.

Dr. Schultz acted disturbed and said, "We're not set at all. After Dr. Kaplan did the nerve root decompressions, his office phoned my office and told them he'd done the operation on you. My office took that to mean he'd done everything that needed to be done and canceled the operating room, the assisting surgeons, the anesthesiologist, and my surgical nurse."

"Oh, no! I want to get it over with and go home! When can we do it?" I asked, badly upset.

"I'll have to go see how soon I can get an operating room and my surgical team rescheduled. I'll come back as soon as I know," he said and left the room hurriedly.

He returned later in the afternoon and said, relieved, "We're set. We have an operating room and everyone's scheduled. We'll do the operation early Saturday morning, three days from now."

How he managed to schedule the orthopedic surgeon to assist, the general surgeon who had done so many of my other operations, my regular surgical nurse, an anesthesiologist, and an operating room on such short notice, especially for a Saturday, I don't know. It was probably like trying to arrange a safari for forty-seven people if you only had one Land Rover: complicated.

Now that the plans were on track again, Dr. Schultz said, "We'll need a myelogram and I've ordered it for this evening. You'll be given an injection of iodine while you're here in your room and then you'll be transferred to a gurney and wheeled to the Radiology Unit for the X rays as soon as they phone your nurse and say they can fit you into their schedule. This particular type of X ray will allow the radiologist and me to check the spinal cord for impingements."

Dr. Schultz had told me a month ago that he'd be doing an anterior spinal fusion this time and that it was "the last house on the block" for me. "If this operation doesn't work, there probably isn't any more surgery that can be done for you." Now he wanted me to understand more about it and said, "I want you to know that this operation is very serious."

"How do you go about it?" I asked.

"When we get you on the operating table, we'll place you on your back and the anesthesiologist will administer the anesthetic with some added solutions, cortisone and potassium for example, and he'll continuously monitor your vital signs as long as you're in surgery. "We'll make an incision at the tip of your hipbone and core out two plugs, dowels, of bone about an inch in diameter. We'll drill a little hole in the center of each one and fit them over a special tool made to hold the plugs in place when we're ready to hammer them into your spine. We'll set them aside until we're ready to use them.

"Next, Dr. Grady, your general surgeon, will open your tummy from above your navel down to your pubic bone. He'll lay open the muscles and move all your organs and arteries aside and fasten them where they'll be out of the way of our work and where they can't get accidentally nicked. That will expose your spinal column from the front so that we can work on it. Our chances of getting a good spinal fusion are better if we work from the front than from the back in patients who've already had previous spinal fusions."

How bizarre, I thought, and envisioned all my innards dangling off the sides of the operating table and held securely out of the way by alligator clips.

Not reading my thoughts (I hoped), Dr. Schultz continued to prepare me for the surgery. "Next, Dr. Hurley and I will go to work cleaning up any fragments and other debris that might be there. When the area is clean, we'll drill a hole between your lumbar-5 and lumbar-6 vertebrae, your trouble spot. The hole will be about an inch in diameter and it will extend from the front of your spine almost to the back, but not quite all the way because a patient can be in serious trouble really fast if there happens to be a slip of the drill and the spinal cord gets damaged."

I cringed. I got the picture. It sounded as though a doctor better know his business well to do this procedure.

"We'll place the plugs from your hipbone into the hole we've made between your vertebrae and hammer them in. I'm really nothing more than a sterile carpenter," he finished modestly.

I didn't buy that at all!

"Do you have any questions?" he asked, determined that I understand what was involved.

There was nothing I needed to ask. Dr. Schultz patted my hand and said, "Then I'll look in on you tomorrow and see how you're doing and early Saturday morning we'll do your operation."

He left me with no illusions. This kind of surgery was going to demand a lot from all of us. I dreaded the operation more than any of the others, yet my back and hip now limited me so much that I couldn't carry on my normal activities. I'd always been a risk taker, one part of me said, so what's so different this time? Why don't I just put myself in the doctor's hands and get on with it? What choice do I have anyway?

Shortly after Dr. Schultz left, the Radiology Unit phoned the nurses' station and said they'd have an opening in their schedule and could take me right away if the nurses would get me ready. The iodine for the myelogram was injected into my arm and within fifteen minutes my face was purplish and I was having another itch attack. Writhing and flailing my arms and legs, I glanced up and saw Wess walking through the doorway unexpectedly.

"What in God's name is wrong with you? I'm going to get a nurse," she cried in alarm and ran out the door.

A nurse hurried in with Benadryl® and gave me an injection, saying sympathetically, "I know you feel terrible, but we have to take you to Radiology now or they won't be able to do the myelogram until tomorrow and that'll be too late."

The nurse and Wess transferred me to a gurney and wheeled me to the elevator. A doctor riding down at the same time watched my crazed scratching and scolded the nurse. "You've got to get her itching controlled! She's tearing up her skin."

"We've given her Benadryl®," the nurse said in self-defense, "but it just hasn't gone to work yet."

The X-ray technicians, already alerted to the reaction, met us and said, "We'll wait with her until the Benadryl® takes effect. She has to be able to hold absolutely still or we can't take the X rays."

Almost as suddenly as the reaction had started, it now diminished enough that if I exerted all my willpower I could stay quiet long enough to have the X rays taken.

"You may have a bad headache from the dye so we want you to drink plenty of water and let your nurse know if you have any kind of problem," a technician said and sent me back upstairs.

Wess stayed with me and bathed my face with cool water while we waited for the nurse to bring a shot to curb the pain in my back. The pain was so bad that a pain cocktail wasn't going to touch it.

"Wess, I'm sorry you had to see one of these reactions," I said to her. "I'm glad you were with me, though. I'm all right now and it's getting dark outside, so I think you should go on home. The security man will walk you to your car if you ask and I'd feel better about you if you did. If you can come back tomorrow, I'll catch you up on everything."

With a worried look she said good night and turned toward the elevator. Her doctor had not yet found a way to bring her blood pressure under control and she didn't need this kind of stress right now; yet, I didn't know of any way to protect her from it. I knew she wouldn't stop coming to help me at a time like this, even for her own health.

March 27 was a get-ready day. Tom came from the store for our daily business conference so that I could give him the last instructions before he took over full responsibility of the store until I could be helpful again or until we sold it. We had end-of-month reports to prepare for the CPAs, sales figures to ana-lyze, businesses to call, and employee schedules to work up. It wasn't fair to put all the work on him, but he didn't hesitate or complain about the long days he was already working or how many more hours he'd be working from now on. We finished our business and I moved ahead to the next thing.

It had been two weeks since my hair had been washed, since no showers were permitted until the incision in my back sealed itself, and it would be another two weeks or more before the next opportunity. I phoned my hairdresser, Sandy Sanchez, and asked her if she could come give me a good shampoo and set.

While we waited, the nurses brought a waterproof wheelchair that had a reclining back and a foot support that raised to make a table I could lie back on with my hair in the shampoo basin. When Sandy arrived, they took me up the hall to a room equipped for shampoos and Sandy gave me a thorough scrub-bing, a conditioner to counteract the drying effect of pillows and sheets, and a fresh hairdo. It probably did more to raise my morale than anything else I could have done.

The Bittners, Wess, and Stanford said they would be available to my mother in case she needed anything during the next few weeks, and I phoned Marilyn Goodsell, the manager of Manzano del Sol, the retirement center where my mother now lived. "Marilyn, this is Mary Zartman's daughter. I'm in the hospital again and I want to give you the phone number for my room; but just in case you can't reach me for some reason, here are the names and numbers of several friends who can help and they'll always be able to find me."

All day long numerous friends came in and out and gave me their love and best wishes. Helen phoned from Las Vegas and Terry phoned from Denver. There were dozens of new flowers and cards full of love and humor and Wess continued her job as keeper of my room.

"I know that you rest the best if your room is clean, organized, and quiet. I just want you to rest. Let me do these things for you," she said when I asked her not to do so much work. She inspected my sleepwear on the IV rack and made sure everything was fresh and clean, reorganized all my other belongings, and showed me where she put each item. She made sure my comb, hand cream, etc., were at my fingertips on the night table.

Stanford came in several times during the day, brought some new cassettes of music, took me for walks in the hall, talked about things other than surgery, and assured me that everything at my empty house was all right. Toward the end of the day everyone else left and Stanford stayed. It was that relatively slack time of evening when the nurses were finished taking patients' vital signs, but it wasn't quite time to serve the evening meals.

Alone together, Stanford and I sat quietly without talking. The time was right for me to tell him some of my feelings. "You've been unbelievably good to me as long as I've known you. I love everything about you and I like to be with you all the time. I want to make you as happy as you make me."

He held my hand and listened as I continued.

"I'm more sorry than I can say that our lives keep being disrupted by these back problems and I want to make it up to you. My promise to you is that I'll use all my energy and I'll fight with all my strength to get well fast. I promise that when I get well I'll build you a very special day, a day to do anything you want to do, wherever you want to do it. Be thinking about what you'd like and where you'd like to go and that's what we'll do."

Eyes soft with love, with no need for words, Stanford nod-
ded his head and smiled with that glow that is uniquely his.
Our embrace was the sealing of my promise and his acceptance.
Our kiss was long and tender as he said good night.

The evening meal was served and later cleared away. Then
Dr. Randy Rosett, the anesthesiologist for this operation, came
to talk with me about what he would be doing and he discussed
with me the medical information that was in my chart. Concerned, sincere, and very pleasant, he reinforced my confidence
in all the medical people who were doing so much to make me
well.

Shortly after Dr. Rosett left, Virginia came to start her pre-op.
"Here we go again. A ten-minute back scrub and a soapy enema.
Aren't we having fun?"

I grimaced at her gallows humor.

"We'll have to take away your carafe of water at midnight and
you can't have anything to eat or drink after that time. If you
want a peanut-butter sandwich or hot spiced cider tonight, let
me fix them before midnight," she offered.

"I would like to have them and whenever you have time to
do it is fine with me," I replied, wanting to be as little a nuisance
as possible.

Virginia prepared the little snack, but I couldn't eat. There
were butterflies in my stomach and I was losing my courage as
the night wore on. It's rare that I ever take a sleeping pill but
this time I welcomed the sedative Virginia brought when she
came to lotion my back, look at the incision to be reopened so
soon, and wish me well.

"I won't be here in the morning when you leave for surgery,
but I'll come see you as soon as I come on duty at five. Till then,
good luck!"

Little did we know . . .

The surgery was early in the morning. At some time that
evening I began to drift in and out of a haze of semiconscious-
ness and knew that I was again in the Advanced Neurological
Unit, Intensive Care.

Bea, Barnett, Wess, and Dee were there throughout the day
waiting for word from the doctors. Stanford came to the

hospital five or six times during the day, but I was always unaccountably still in surgery.

Finally I was out of surgery, out of the recovery room, and in a room where he was allowed to come in and see me. It was comforting to see his face even if I wasn't awake enough to talk with him. It was enough just to know he was there.

In this Intensive Care Unit a nurse was with me every moment. There were no phone calls, no flowers, and no visitors, except for those few people who were closest to me and even they were only allowed to come in one at a time and very briefly.

During the first endless night I rose and sank in scalding whirlpools of pain. Injections of painkiller didn't come often enough or last long enough to help. Nurses rolled me from side to side every two hours and I wept at the brutality of it. "Please, please don't hurt me anymore," I begged. So this was Intensive Care, the best care they could give?

Morning came and Dr. Schultz and Dr. Grady made their rounds. I heard their conversation with the nurses and listened to the pages of my chart turning in the silent room before they came to stand beside my bed. "Good morning! How do you feel?"

"Like hell!" I wanted to say, but my mouth was so dry and my throat ached from the tube running up my nostril and down the back of my throat, making it impossible to breathe through my nose or swallow. Oh, for some water! And a toothbrush!

Dr. Grady checked the IV bottles hanging on the racks and the solutions dripping down the tubes and through the needles into my hands. He looked at the drainage tube that ran from my tummy and the catheter from my bladder.

Dr. Schultz said quietly, "Your spine was worse than we expected when we got a good look at it and we ran into a lot of problems we hadn't been able to foresee. We knew you had one joint that needed to be fused, but when we got a clear view of your spine, we found you had two levels that needed to be fused instead. With two fusions we needed more bone plugs, so we had to open both your hips rather than one, and core out four plugs, not two. It was hard to get enough bone because we'd already taken two plugs out of your right hip for a previous fusion and we'd shaved staves of bone off it for another one."

He hesitated but had more to say. "Another problem was that we couldn't get one of your major arteries moved away from your vertebrae so we couldn't drill our hole straight into the spine. We had to drill from an awkward, hard-to-reach angle, and hammer in the plug from a bad angle, too. When you see your next X rays, you'll see a lot of little stainless-steel clips still fastened to your veins. We had to sever a goodly number of veins and seal them with the clips, but they can be left inside permanently without causing any problem."

A pause, a deep breath, and the doctor continued. "Another problem was that we couldn't get one of your major arteries to stop bleeding and had to give you several transfusions. We used all of the units of A-Negative blood you had self-donated and then took extra units from the blood bank. Finally we ran out of time for safely working on your body and had to get out in a hurry before it caused problems of another kind."

So that's why I feel so bad, I thought. I have an incision in my back, an incision down half of my front, and an incision in each hip. Dowels of bone have been drilled out of both hip-bones. Three vertebrae have been scraped, have had holes drilled in them, and have had plugs an inch wide hammered into the holes. I'm full of steel clips and staples and empty of blood. There are tubes in my nose and throat, needles and tubes in both arms, and tubes in my stomach and bladder. My nostrils burn, my throat aches, and my head is about to split. I can barely croak when I try to talk, but who cares? I don't have anything to say anyway.

I was in blazing agony.

Throughout the day teams of nurses came to my bed to grasp the drawsheet, roll my body, and block it in place with pillows. The pain of being touched, let alone moved, was unbearable and when they turned me on my side, it felt as though all the incisions in my body were ripping apart from the strain of flesh pulling away as my body weight settled onto one hip. The pain was excruciating. It even hurt to breathe.

I tried to clear my foggy head and remember enough physiology to understand why just the simple act of taking a breath made the hip pain so horrendous. I discovered that the less I breathed, the less badly it hurt my hips, and I finally succeeded in barely breathing at all. There! That was better!

Gradually I became vaguely aware of nurses paging my doctors. Was somebody sick?

Dr. Grady rushed into the room, looked at me, and quickly called the Respiratory Unit. A technician hurried in with a breathing device. "Blow into this tube," I was told. "Make the disc in the cylinder rise to this mark. You have to clear those lungs."

I tried but I couldn't force any air into it. Dr. Grady called Radiology for an X-ray unit to take a picture of my chest.

"She has a collapsed lung," the technician said.

"Get your equipment over here and get her breathing! Start her on this medication to break up the congestion!"

Despite the flurry surrounding me, I didn't seem to be any part of it. I was strangely outside, looking on, and not even especially interested. The only thing that was real was the torment of raging pain. Now and then the fog of pain would clear enough for me to see someone standing by my bed and sometimes, but only if they told me their names, I could remember that they were my best friends.

Dody, my friend for fifteen years, now seemed like a kind lady whose name I thought I ought to know but couldn't remember. She watched me briefly and marched out to the nurses' station. Appalled and distressed at how I looked, she scolded the nurses about my misery. "Isn't there something you can do for her?!" she shouted.

The nurses answered solemnly, "We know she's suffering and we're doing everything we can."

Morning after morning the nurses told me Terry had phoned from Denver to ask how I was and give me his love. They said flowers were still arriving, but they couldn't bring them inside the room, so they'd put them right outside the door till I could have them.

Lab technicians came perpetually to draw a syringe or two or three of blood. What's left? I wondered.

Doctors came and went throughout the day.

I wasn't getting any food, but with that tube down my throat, I didn't care even though my bones seemed to be sticking out of my skin. My bowels didn't function and I was uncomfortable.

One of the nurses in the haze asked a doctor if she couldn't at least take the tube out of my nose and throat and give me that much relief, but the doctor said she absolutely could not, not until my bowels began making sounds of activity or I'd blow up and hurt even more.

Another night was coming on. How many had there been? Eight? Nine? I tried to remember how long I'd been in Intensive Care. I was so tired and my misery was so total, so absolute, that I couldn't stand it anymore. I just wanted to be dead. I was barely breathing anyway and all I'd have to do was just stop. It would be so easy to die. Now.

I gathered what was left of my last ounce of strength to call the nurse and give her a message for Stanford, but something stopped me. In that final moment of despair, some small portion of my mind that was still sane reminded me that I'd made a promise to Stanford that I'd fight with all my strength to get well quickly and build him a very special day to make up for all of this. Suddenly I realized how cruel it would be for a stranger to say to Stanford, the greatest love of my life, "Excuse me, Mr. Hall, wait a minute! I have a message for you. Lucy said to tell you she's sorry, but she won't be building you that special day she promised you. She got tired of all the trying to get well and she just quit."

I shuddered.

And took another breath.

Chapter 14

TURNING THE CORNER

One by one the needles and tubes were removed from my body and it began to resume its functions without the help of intravenous solutions, extra medications, and specialized equipment. My mind cleared enough that I recognized friends, talked coherently with doctors and nurses, and once again participated in my own care.

For the first time in nine days I became aware that my hair was uncombed and tangled and it felt dirty. My teeth hadn't been brushed for the same length of time and only the lemon-flavored swabs that Stanford had run over my teeth and in my mouth in Intensive Care had given me any relief from the thirst, dryness, and bad taste. I felt ugly and tired.

Embarrassed at being such a mess, I tried to console myself with thoughts like this: if they took away Elizabeth Taylor's polished nails, eyelashes, makeup, and hairdo, and ran all of the same tubes and needles into her that were in me, I bet no one would be able to tell us apart. It wasn't really consoling though. Elizabeth Taylor had already had more than her share of medical catastrophes and she was probably gorgeous through all of them.

The nurses now gave me sponge baths and rubbed lotion on my skin, dry and flaking from medications and weeks of lying on sheets. With the greatest of care they turned me from one

side of the bed to the other and put fresh linens on the mat-
tress. It was heavenly to feel so clean.

Dr. Grady came to talk with me and look at the incisions.
"You've lost a lot of blood and you've lost a lot of weight. That's
part of the reason you feel so tired. You need a nutritious diet
and supplemental high-nutrition drinks to rebuild your
strength, gain some weight, and make your bones grow. There
are several kinds of supplemental drinks that are loaded with
vitamins and minerals and I'm going to order them for you to
drink four times a day. I'll ask the dietary supervisor to drop by
and tell you more about them and I want her to help you plan
your menus for the highest nutrition."

Every time Dr. Grady had come to see me he had been so
kind and warm, so attentive to any complaint I had, and so thorough in treating each ailment that I had become very fond of
him. I trusted him completely.

The nutritionist, slender, energetic, and the picture of good
health, came to my room later in the morning. "Let's talk about
the supplemental drinks Dr. Grady's ordered for you and you
can choose the flavors you like. They all taste good, especially
over ice, and you'll like drinking them. Then let's talk about the
kinds of foods that are going to be best for rebuilding your body
and we'll make out your menus."

The nutritionist gave me a short course on vitamins and minerals and we began to select my meals for the next two days. It
was a surprise to me that such a large and busy institution would
provide a number of foods that weren't on the menu at all, but
that a patient could receive just by writing them on the order.

During the second week after the surgery I rested, read, and
slept. The pain was terribly bad, but it was made more bearable
by the shots of Benadryl® first, and ten minutes later the
painkiller. The nurses, working in pairs, used the drawsheet to
turn my body regularly, but it was no longer as awful as it had
been.

Since I was still flat on my back, I ate my meals lying down. I
tried to keep gelatin dessert—which I couldn't see on the tray
above me—on a spoon and guide it into my mouth, but I finally
resorted to eating it like finger food. I tried to sip soup through
a straw without scalding myself or pouring it down my neck.

Stanford often came at lunchtime to help me manage and Wess came in the evening to cut my food into small bites and hand it to me. Mealtime became easier once my head was raised enough that I could see what I was doing.

Every day the nurses raised the head of the bed a little higher than the day before and gradually increased it to about forty degrees as my sore tummy, hips, and back tolerated the movement better.

During the second week Dr. Hester dropped by to say hello each day but didn't stay to tire me with conversation. Physical therapy was also suspended.

At about the tenth day after the anterior spinal fusion, Dr. Schultz approved my gains and said, "Today it's time to get you up. I'll have the nurses come in and help you sit up on the edge of the bed and dangle your feet over the side. You're going to do that several times a day for two or three days and then they'll stand you on your feet and start you walking again. It will hurt but I want you to do it anyway."

The nurses came to show me the technique to sitting up. "First, press the electric bed control and raise the head of your bed until you're sitting up. Now, reach this arm across in front of your body and place your hand on the side of the bed for support while you use your other elbow and forearm to raise your body. We're going to gently lift your feet and move them over the side of the bed so they dangle and we'll help you support your upper body in a sitting position," they explained.

It *did* hurt! My back, hips, and tummy screamed at the pressures exerted on them and the nurses quickly and gently laid me back in bed. Never would it hurt that much again! How had Ted Kitchel been able to move so well so fast? I wondered.

Three days at the hard work of sitting up and dangling my feet gave me the confidence to move ahead, and when Dr. Schultz wrote the orders for me to stand up with the assistance of the nurses and take a few steps with the walker, I was prepared. I thought. When I stood up and all of my weight had to be borne by my beaten-up spine, however, I shrieked at the violence of the pain that was beyond belief. I didn't want to act like a baby, but the pain was terrible! My determined resolution always had been that no matter how hard it is to do something the doctor tells me to do, I'll say out loud to him, "I do want to do it and I will try." Now, however, that resolution was difficult to uphold.

"The first time is the hardest," the nurses comforted me. "We'll help you do it again this afternoon and you'll see that it won't be as bad."

I could hardly wait!

The physical therapists resumed assisting me to use the walker properly. They worked to increase my endurance for walking, taught me to turn around in such a way that I didn't twist my back or lose my balance, and helped me walk with a more even gait.

Every morning Dr. Schultz, Dr. Grady, and Dr. Mitchell came to talk with me, review my medications, make adjustments in the dosages, and inspect my incisions. At last, after about two weeks, the day I was waiting for was finally here. The incisions had sealed themselves, there were no unhealed openings, and the staples could be removed. That meant I could take a shower and shampoo!

Sally was my nurse that morning and saw how excited I was about getting to take a shower. She brought a waterproof wheelchair that had a hole in the seat, gathered my soap, shampoo, toothbrush, and toothpaste, and wheeled me up the hall to a shower room so big the whole Dallas Cowboys team could shower there.

The warm spray gave me the same exuberance that a baby elephant must feel when it finally reaches a lake and his mother turns her shower hose on him. I sprayed, soaped, shampooed, rinsed, sprayed some more, brushed, and gurgled, and could have easily stayed all day. I couldn't bend over or reach up or back, but I could bathe my face, arms, and body, and Sally sudsed my back and legs. I was clean—really clean! It was a whole new world!

The nurses took me for walks whenever they could spare a few minutes and Sally regularly helped me during the mornings, but she still didn't like the scuffs I used and I hadn't sent for any others. "I'm not at all happy with those slippers! You can slip them on without bending over, but they don't give your foot any support. The muscles in your foot and ankle are still so weak that your foot can fold up at any time and cause you to fall. You need a slipper that holds your foot more securely! When are you going to get some?"

Virginia, my nurse during the afternoons and evenings, also went to great lengths to help me correct a problem with the way I walked. For many months before the operations, my back and hip hurt so badly that I compensated for it by turning my right foot outward about forty-five degrees and that caused my balance to shift and affected my gait.

Now that the nerve damage was corrected, Dr. Schultz directed me to retrain that foot. "I want you to point your toes directly in front of you and step down firmly. Don't let those toes turn to the side and stop favoring that leg. It puts strain on your spinal fusion."

I didn't believe I could change the way I walked. My back and hip didn't hurt as much if I walked with my foot turned out and I limped because that side hurt more than the other side. Besides, it was a habit by now and habits are hard to break. My progress in improving my gait was slow and discouraging and my attitude was only half-hearted. The muscles and tendons that had been doing all the work weren't the ones I needed now and the ones I did need were lazy.

Virginia took me for a walk in the halls late one night before she went off duty and observed critically the placement of each step. She asked me kindly to correct it.

"I'm trying, but I can't. I forget," I argued.

Not affected she said simply, "All you have to do is remember to point that toe straight ahead of you one step at a time."

"One step at a time" was an increment I could deal with, but walking straight for a whole lifetime was not. For just one step I could try.

During the next six weeks, I trained myself to be conscious of every step I took and laboriously forced myself to lift the foot, turn it to a straightened position, and set it down firmly; and for four months beyond that, it was still necessary to pay attention to my foot and concentrate on carrying my body evenly with every step. It was tiresome and boring but it worked. Eventually my feet moved parallel to each other and my gait became fluid.

Chapter 15

HOME FOR EASTER

After two weeks my doctors believed I was strong enough to resume daily conversations with the psychologist, Dr. Hester. He knew throughout this time what was happening and how bad it got, so I was puzzled when he sat down beside me, now that it was all in the past, and said, "Now the hard part begins."

"What do you mean? I've gone through the worst of it and from now on everything will be better," I countered.

"The hard part begins now because it's time for you to discard many of your old attitudes and behaviors and learn new ones. You'll have to accept certain limitations and learn to make accommodations for them. Your work, your recreation, your social activities, and the way you take care of your health will all have to change."

It made me tired to think about it.

Dr. Hester continued, "Your doctors, nurses, and physical therapists are evaluating your progress in view of determining when you can go home. They want to be sure you're making steady progress, be certain that your medications are in balance, and be as secure as they can be that you won't have any troublesome setbacks at home alone. I want to feel confident that you can make the emotional adjustment from being in a hospital where you are surrounded with health care and the company of other people to being at home in an empty, two-story house with no assistance."

"I don't have to be alone all the time," I said. "Stanford said he'd come over every morning and make breakfast and drop by on his way home from work each evening to see if I needed anything."

"What about the rest of the day? What arrangements can you make for care? What will you do if you have an emergency at night?" Dr. Hester asked.

He made it clear that I'd have to get some help for a few weeks and convinced me to accept the offers of friends to come over during each day to check on me. I hated to impose or lean on them, but Dr. Hester led me to look at it from the other side. "Suppose this was your friend Wess who was going home to an empty house with no care waiting and she refused your offers to help. How would you feel about the quality of your friendship?"

We listed what my daily needs were going to be and there wasn't any question that I needed to hire a housekeeper who could help me, so I set about locating several women and interviewing them by telephone. A couple of days later I said to Dr. Hester, "I've hired a housekeeper to come in for four hours a day for one month. She'll keep house, do the laundry, buy the groceries, run errands, and take me to the doctors' appointments. With her help, with my friends, and with Stanford, I should be all right. Do you think I can go home for Easter?" I was as prepared as I could be to make the transition from the hospital with its constant care to home and my friends, and although I had some anxiety about being on my own, I could hardly wait to regain some privacy in my life.

"I've signed your release," Dr. Schultz said soon afterward. My other doctors approved it and I prepared to leave the hospital. I'd miss everyone and I'd miss their care.

On the thirty-seventh day of hospitalization, Wess and Stanford came to pack my belongings and take me home. Wess had been at the hospital every day to keep my belongings neat, take my lingerie to launder, encourage me to do all the things that doctors and nurses said would help me get well, and sometimes bring a Mexican dinner as a change from hospital food. Now as Wess packed my clothes, one of the nurses who had seen her there day after day said admiringly, "I wish I had a friend like you. I think I'll start looking now so that if I ever get sick I'll have someone to help me like you helped Lucy."

Wess took some of my things to her car and drove to my house to meet Bea and Barnett.

The hospital business office prepared the release papers for my signature, and Darlene and Sally brought the sheet of instructions from the doctor. They began to read the instructions to me with Stanford listening so that he'd know them too.

"Dr. Schultz says you're not to do any bending, lifting, or reaching. Do no driving. Do no prolonged sitting or standing. You can have sex as tolerated. Diet is as prescribed," and so on.

I did a double take, sure I'd heard wrong, and said, "Go back. What did you just say about sex? Are you reading that or making it up?" I knew full well that they were especially capable of making up anything to tease Stanford.

"'Sex as tolerated' is what it says," Sally said, pointing to it on the sheet of instructions.

Ah! Things were getting better!

I had already read in books and articles about back problems that sex is good for the back whether the back is healthy or recuperating, and a person's good sense can tell him if a particular position for making love is too stressful. If it is, there are plenty of other ways to go about it. It's important to any back patient to release tension, since it lessens back pain, and good sex does that as well as providing plenty of other benefits, too.

The nurses left the room for a moment to see other patients and I said to Stanford, "I'm really sorry that my back has interrupted our love life. I can hardly wait to get home and get better."

Stanford looked at me very directly with a bright sparkle in his eyes and wryly stated, "That's all right. *Too* much sex is like the dry heaves. You go through all the motions but nothing happens." He left the room to take my suitcase to the car.

The nurses came hurrying back into the room to find out what was so funny, but all they saw was a respected businessman carrying my suitcase toward the elevator and a back patient in convulsions of laughter.

It would be fun to be home again!

What should have been a simple task, riding from the hospital to home, was exhausting, even though Stanford and Wess did all the work of packing, carrying my things, and driving.

Bea and Barnett went to my house at midmorning to meet the new housekeeper and show her through the rooms and storage closets where cleaning supplies and equipment were kept. They had the house warm and ready when we got there.

My new town house, still not entirely finished, was one I was proud of, but it was now a problem, too. A two-story home, the living room, dining room, sun-room, kitchen, and a three-quarter bathroom were on the ground floor, while the bedrooms, closets, and full bathrooms were on the second floor, thirteen steps up—thirteen steps I couldn't climb.

There was a choice: settle on the ground floor, or settle on the second floor and stay there until I had the muscle strength and steadiness to climb up and down the stairs safely. If I chose to live upstairs for a few weeks, I wouldn't be able to prepare any of my meals or answer the front door. On the other hand, if I decided to live downstairs, any clothing, bedding, or other things from the closets or dressers would have to be brought downstairs. Also, the controls for the heating and air-conditioning system were at the top of the stairs, and at this time of year, we had cold nights but hot days and needed both systems.

We talked it over and decided that I should build my nest downstairs and each day make a list of items I needed from upstairs. Whoever happened to be there would bring them down. What did people with bad backs in truly large houses in the East and Midwest do? I wondered. Surely they don't all have elevators or chair lifts.

Stanford, knowing how badly I wanted to be able to do things for myself, wanted a guarantee that I wouldn't attempt to climb the stairs before my body was strong enough and he exacted a promise from me. "Promise me you won't go up the stairs if I'm not here," he said one morning after breakfast.

Agreeably I answered, "Okay."

"That won't be good enough when you think you need something from upstairs and you don't want to wait for anyone to come over and get it for you. Say, 'I promise.'"

I raised my right hand and stated in a loud, smart-aleck voice to my in-house attorney, "I promise I will not go up the stairs if you're not here," and had my impudence answered by his "heaven help me" look.

The promise did keep me on the ground floor a number of times when the temptation to do things for myself was stronger than my body was.

We made my bed on the new, extralong, creamy leather sofa and I slept there as well as I would have slept anywhere, as tender and aching as I was. I used the walker to go to the kitchen for a glass of milk or water, but I couldn't stand up long enough to cook. I ate peanut-butter sandwiches and fruit and drank high-nutrition milk drinks. Friends often brought wonderful special little meals in the evenings.

In general, the system of listing items to be carried up or down the stairs worked well. There was one day, however, when I forgot to ask anyone to turn off the air conditioner or bring down a nightgown and blanket. As the desert temperature dropped, the air conditioner made the house colder and colder and, with no blanket, I finally crawled underneath the leather sofa cushions and stayed curled up there until Stanford came over for breakfast and found me icy and miserable. On another day I forgot to ask that my pain pills be brought down and I went much too long with no relief from the hurting. I was a basket case by the time someone came to look in on me. Most of my misery was caused by my own negligence in planning what I'd need later, and to make a mistake once was enough to force me to pay attention and not let it happen again.

At the hospital, when I'd interviewed housekeepers by telephone, the one who seemed especially interested in the job told me she had years of experience caring for convalescents and knew all about what to do. I hired her and knew I'd depend on her for considerable help. After a couple of days of her help, however, I had serious questions about my choice. The woman did the laundry all right, but when she put things away, she put them where she thought they should go, not where I told her to put them, and there are items of clothing I still haven't found.

She went through all the motions of cleaning, humming as she worked, but when she finished, the sinks weren't clean and the counters had crumbs on them. I asked her to clean the winter film off the front windows and she did that, but she left the screens lying in the shrubbery.

If someone telephoned, she answered the phone but laid it down and forgot to tell me. If I called someone myself, that's when she started to vacuum in the same room. She made it difficult for me to walk around by leaving cleaning equipment and electrical cords in the middle of the hallway where I couldn't get past them with the walker. She made me so nervous and aggravated that I could hardly be civil. That kind of help was causing me more stress than I could handle and I didn't know what to do: keep her and continue trying to train her or terminate her and not have any help at all.

The dilemma solved itself before long. About an hour before she was to finish for the day I said, "Before you leave today, I want you to be sure and polish the pedestal bases on the dining table and chairs." She nodded in understanding, but instead of doing it, she fiddle-faddled around doing no work at all. Fifteen minutes before time for her to leave, unable to stand it any longer, I said, "Aren't you going to polish those pedestals?"

She looked at me as though I had a warped sense of priorities and answered, "I can't do it today. It's almost time for my bingo game and I can't concentrate on cleaning."

That was the last straw! I told her I'd have to let her go and she said to me, sounding relieved, "That's all right. I'll be sure to be in time for bingo if I leave now."

Well, she's gone, but where in the world will I find a good, honest housekeeper by tomorrow? I moaned to myself when she left. I called several friends, got a few names from them, and began phoning women. One young woman was especially highly recommended, and when I phoned her, I realized that the name was the same as the one who had been most strongly recommended to me last winter when I was looking for a new seamstress for the store. It was shortly afterwards that I had to leave the store, so I hadn't gotten to meet her or hire her.

I asked her to come over to see the house and talk about becoming my housekeeper. A short time later I answered the doorbell and was surprised to see a beautiful, pale, serene young woman with almond eyes, dressed in the white clothing, leggings, and turban of a Sikh. She stepped into the living room, holding the hands of two little children, and introduced herself.

"I'm Sarb Sarang Kaur Khalsa and these are my twin sons," she said and presented two cute, quiet, mannerly little boys finished with school for the day.

I showed her the house, we discussed the amount of help I needed, and agreed on her schedule and salary. She would start tomorrow!

That was the best thing that could have happened to me. Sarb Sarang, educated and cultured and conscientious about her work, became a good dear friend who helped make me well.

My house well taken care of, I slept on the sofa for three weeks and longed for my big waterbed and for deep, warm, bubble baths upstairs. One morning Stanford said, "I think you should do everything for yourself that you can safely do and do nothing that can hurt you. Do you want to try to climb the stairs tomorrow?"

"Do I! I want to go up and down the stairs whenever I feel like it!" I said excitedly.

"All right. When I come over to make breakfast tomorrow, I'll help you climb the stairs. I'll cover your vanity chair with a plastic bag and put it in the shower so you can sit down to shower and shampoo and stay in it for as long as you want to. The doctor said you can't have tub baths yet, but you might like taking showers until you can have your bubble baths."

All night I kept waking up in delicious anticipation. I hadn't had a real shower for more than a month. I'm going to stay in it all day, I dreamed.

Stanford arrived for breakfast and watched me as I used the walker to reach the foot of the stairs. Then, hitching up my gown and robe to keep from tripping on them, I placed one foot on the bottom step. With both hands pulling hard on the railing and Stanford lifting me at my waist, I raised myself to place my weight on my stronger foot and drew the other foot upward. The moment that all of my weight went onto one foot alone, the other foot in midair, pain ripped through my hip and back so badly that I trembled and broke out in perspiration, and tears of pain ran down my face.

Determined to climb to the top and get that coveted shower, I stepped up once again. The pain was as fierce that time as it was before. I stepped up once again, and again, and again.

It took an eternity, it seemed, to reach the top of the stairs and step into the hot shower I wanted so much. The water sprayed over my face and mixed with my tears of pain and of happiness. I was filled with deep gratitude for this small yet colossal success and for Stanford's patience with me. "Tomorrow," I assured him, "it will be easier."

Spring turned into summer and my strength grew while the pain diminished. During the third month after surgery, Dr. Schultz said I had enough muscle strength to drive the car. I could hardly wait to take my first drive.

I did have one concern, however. When I was in the hospital I had some trouble with vertigo, but I thought little of it. Problems were all relative and that was comparatively minor. The vertigo worsened steadily, however, and was now so bad that I got dizzy enough just sitting or standing to lose my balance and fall over. If I were lying in bed and turned over, I couldn't stop my head from spinning dizzily.

I made my own diagnosis, of course, and told Stanford it was an inner-ear infection. I said I thought I should stay off the stairs and should not drive the car until it cleared up. He took me to an ear specialist.

"My initial diagnosis," the doctor said after an examination, "is that you have a neuroma on the nerve in your inner ear. If further tests confirm it, we'll need to remove the neuroma surgically."

When I heard "surgically," I froze. I didn't even ask what he was talking about.

Further studies showed that there was not a neuroma, however. "You have considerable swelling in your ear. I don't know why it's there, but I want you to decrease your salt intake and increase the amount of water you drink. See me again in a week," the doctor said.

At home I thought about it. My inner ear was swollen and, now that I paid attention, I saw that my hands, feet, and ankles were also swollen. Then the answer struck me. Two months ago my doctor had reduced my dosage of diuretics used to counter the water-retentive effects of cortisone in order to conserve the potassium in my body. I was still taking the minimum dosage.

I did something I wouldn't normally do and never recommend. I dashed as fast as I could in a walker to the medicine closet, got the diuretics, and put myself back on the normal dosage. Within three days all the swelling was gone from my hands, feet, and ankles, and the vertigo had disappeared completely. I was stable.

"I can drive!" I yelled to my empty house and gathered my billfold and keys. My first drive was only around the block, where I could test my muscle strength and reaction time. I did great!

"Tomorrow," I said aloud to myself, "I'm going for a real drive! Pretty soon I'll be doing more things for myself and I won't have to depend so much on other people. I'm going to whip this thing yet!"

Chapter 16

YOU'LL THINK YOU'RE
SUPERWOMAN AGAIN

It's not what you say; it's what I hear that counts.

L. M. D.

Any small reason was an excuse for me to get into the car and drive. I loved being out in the sunny weather, seeing which buildings and businesses were new, meshing with the traffic on the freeways, and cruising the winding hilly streets at the foot of the mountains overlooking the green valley and the city.

There were some limitations as to where I could do my shopping, errands, and banking, and it took a few trips to learn about them. For instance, if a business didn't have handicap parking, I didn't have enough endurance to walk from a more distant parking space and couldn't do business there. If the doors on a building were very heavy, I didn't have the muscle strength to pull them open and my back was still too tender to wrench the doors open with a jerk. Some doors had such tight springs that they slammed shut before I could get the walker and myself through them and I'd gotten caught between the steel door and the frame more than once. I'd badly cut the back of my heel in one of the mishaps.

Never before had I understood the problems of the handicapped or paid any attention to their campaigns to make city, state, and federal governments more responsive to their physical requirements. For the first time I learned the importance of handicap license plates. My viewpoint shifted dramatically now that I had one myself.

Sarb Sarang bought my groceries regularly, but I was eager to do as many of my own tasks as I could, especially grocery shopping. I'd always liked to look at all the new products and take them home to try, so it would be fun and good for me, I figured, to begin shopping for myself. I was ready to test my ability to do it. I was sure that if I asked the store manager to keep my walker while I pushed a grocery cart, the cart could be my support. I wondered if a manager would be good-natured about it or grumpy at the inconvenience. How far would I be able to walk before the back and hip pain became too fierce to continue? Would I have to stand in a long check-out line, and could I do that? I wouldn't know until I tried.

My goal for the first shopping trip was modest, I thought. I'd drive to the supermarket and park near the door, unload the walker and walk into the store, use a grocery cart for support long enough to find just five items, check out with the cashier, carry the groceries to the car, drive home, and put away the groceries. What a change from all those years of dashing in and out of stores without a thought!

I chose one of the smaller supermarkets for the test, drove up, parked, walked in, and asked the manager, "Do you have a place where I can leave my walker while I shop, please?"

Courteously, he stored the walker at his own desk and brought me a grocery cart. So far, so good.

Supported by the cart, I walked through enough of the store to find four of the items on the list, but by then I was in too much pain and was too exhausted to look for the fifth item. There was a short line at the check-out and waves of dizziness and nausea washed over me as I shifted my weight from leg to leg and leaned on the cart trying to bear the paralyzing pain in my back and hips. At last the clerk checked me out and I went to the car. For a long while I sat there shaking from exhaustion and sobbing from pain, unable to drive out onto the streets. I was disappointed and depressed that I still had so far to go before I was well.

During the next two weeks I built my strength and endurance

by walking up and down the stairs, doing isometric exercises, and going for walks on the driveway. The first day I only walked to the house next door before I had to turn around and go back home. The second day I was able to reach the third house and by the end of two weeks I was strong enough to walk to the end of the block and back with the walker. I was ready for another test at the grocery store.

The afternoon temperature was ninety-three degrees and I put on cool, white tennis shorts and shirt and drove to the same store as before. The manager traded a grocery cart for my walker and I began to shop for the items on the list. I stopped at the deli counter for some sliced roast beef, and while I was standing there, a nice-looking, well-dressed man stopped beside me, looked me up and down, and said, "Excuse me, but how do you stay so good-looking?"

Astonished and more flattered than I wanted to admit, I fibbed, "Oh, I work out all the time," and thanked him. What a change in attitude that stranger created! He didn't seem to look at me as being ill or handicapped, so maybe nobody else would either. I decided I'd try harder than ever to get well and look as normal as I used to look.

While I was in the hospital, Dr. Hester spent an hour a day with me working on my counterproductive attitudes and my compulsion to drive myself beyond endurance. Now I drove to his office for a one-hour conference every week and he did much to help me. Nevertheless, I asked to quit seeing him, at least for a period of time.

"My medical bills are at $40,000 already, not counting yours. My insurance companies are still reviewing the bills, they haven't paid any of them, and I don't have any way of knowing how many they are going to pay. I'm afraid to run up any more expenses."

Dr. Hester said, "Let's not worry about that right now. You're doing beautifully, but I'm afraid that if you stop coming now you'll go back to thinking you're Superwoman and can do anything. You can't, and I need to make sure you can deal with that fact. Let's keep working and I'll let you know if I hear anything about your insurance claims."

Still worried, but knowing I did still need help, I agreed to continue.

"I want you to buy a book that will give you more of an understanding of yourself. It's called *The Superwoman Syndrome,* by Marjorie Hansen Shaevitz. Read it this week and we'll talk about it when you come back the next time."

He was right. It was a revelation to me. I was caught up in trying to be a Superwoman and I didn't even know there was any other way to live. I'd been that way all my life and so had everyone else in my family. It might have helped all of us to get ahead in life, but in my case it backfired. For some reason I didn't seem to have the physical constitution to keep the pace forever. Had I worn out my body from overextending myself, I wondered, or was I just the runt of the litter?

"You don't have to know everything and do everything, and it's okay to be poor at doing some of the things you try to do. You're allowed to have weaknesses and you're allowed to make mistakes. You can stop punishing yourself for having warts," Dr. Hester assured me.

Looking at myself as an outside observer would, I said, "It would be easier for other people around me if I stopped driving myself so hard and expecting perfection of myself, wouldn't it?"

"Yes. From what you've told me, you don't expect any of your employees or friends to be perfect or to push themselves beyond their limits and you aren't disappointed in them for not doing it. Don't you see that they'll feel the same way about you if you relax a little of the pressure toward yourself?"

Dr. Hester talked with me about another aspect of my behavior that was working against me and that I needed to change. "You only have two gears: all or nothing. When you decide to do something, you make up your mind to do all of it, do it right, and do it now. You want it all. Then, when you accomplish most of your goal, always at a high level of excellence except perhaps for some small segment that wasn't as perfect as you wanted it to be, you think you failed with the entire project. You think you did nothing right. Life isn't the same as a feasibility study for a business. You don't have to prove to a board of directors that a project you're considering will either be a complete success or a complete failure and either begin the project or scuttle it based on the prediction. In life you can allow yourself some success and also some failure. It's normal.

You're missing out on some fine experiences by refusing to go for partial rewards when you think you can't have them all."

In other sessions we worked on my should/ought syndrome.

"You keep making yourself feel guilty by not being physically able to do what you think you should or ought to be able to do. You told me, 'I ought to be able to do all of my own grocery shopping by now.' Says who? You said, 'It's been three months since the last operation and I should be able to work.' Why should you be able? If all of your battery of doctors say your bones aren't solid, what makes you think you should meet some invisible timetable for a mold you can't fit?"

He was right again. It was part of my pattern and I frequently used "should" and "ought" in my conversations. Now that I looked at it objectively, it was ridiculous.

Another area Dr. Hester helped me with was to accept that I do have a bad back.

"This is only a temporary condition that I'm going to get partly over at least. I'm not ready to give up trying to get over it and to get my old, normal way of life back again," I argued.

"You have to accept that you have certain limitations that will remain with you for the rest of your life and you must learn new ways to compensate for them," the psychologist insisted forcefully.

"Well, how can I know for sure that I won't ever be able to do some of these things I've always done and want to do again?" I asked, needing a clear answer.

"I would say that after all of your years of back treatments, almost every test known to orthopedic medicine, eleven back procedures done in eight separate operations, and an unknown number of specialists, you can accept it as a fact that you have a crummy back and you're going to have a crummy back for the rest of your life," he replied.

That was a clear enough answer! For the first time ever my mind moved toward looking at my condition realistically: I have a crummy back.

"All right," I capitulated. "I'll change the way I live but I don't know how to start. What do I do?"

During the next several weeks we explored the areas of work in which I could use my training and experience but at the same time stay within the limits of my physical capabilities. It wasn't going to be easy to fit into the working world this time, especially because of my physical limitations and the frequent and extended illnesses that were not even related to my back. Personnel managers frown on employees who ask for time off work two or three times a week to see a doctor and anyone who was interested in me was going to need to know how unsteady an employee I've been for several years. I really didn't want to start a business of my own again, either, and take the risk of having the same thing happen that had happened with the store.

Dr. Hester worked with me to learn how to pace myself. He had me keep logs of how much time I spent doing any single activity, how my body reacted to it, and what modifications I needed to make in order to protect my body from too much stress. He taught me to alternate my activities among sitting, standing, and walking, and to intersperse them with periods of time lying down.

He monitored my records of pain and the number of painkillers I took and made me see the direct relationship between too much stress and too much pain. The records were clear: when I took appropriate care of my body, I needed fewer painkillers; when I fell into my old habits of high stress, the pain soared. Up to a point, control of pain was up to me.

I bought a copy of *Mind Over Back Pain,* by John Sarno, M.D., and found ideas there that I could use to control my pain too.

The social season was in full swing and two of the invitations I received caused a real dilemma for me. I wasn't used to looking like a handicapped person and I was embarrassed at using a walker and wearing flat shoes. I still couldn't stand up for any length of time, and crowds and noise made me tired and nervous. I especially wanted to go to two of the parties, however.

One of them was a reception at the Albuquerque Country Club for Mark Medoff, the playwright, whose *Children of a Lesser God* was playing everywhere. Mark and his family were friends of my brother Dave and his family so I wanted to relay their regards, and since I hadn't seen Mark since a party a year ago, I looked forward to talking with him and congratulating him on his newest success. Mark was able to handle the themes of physical and emotional conditions so sensitively that his plays and films were truly consciousness-raising works. I wished he would write a drama about bad backs and the emotional effect of them.

The other invitation was for a barbecue and swim party at Gail Hollinger and her husband's new home at Tanoan Country Club. Gail was one of our top models for the store, beautiful and multitalented, and her husband was an orthopedic surgeon whom I'd not had an opportunity to meet. Their party was for patrons of the opera and I wanted to see friends who would be there, but I especially wanted to see Gail and meet her husband.

I talked to Dr. Hester about the parties. "I want to go but I don't know how much standing and walking I'll have to do. None of the people who'll be there have ever seen me in flat shoes or a walker. What will they think when they see me? What if I get tired faster than I expect and have to leave so early that I'm conspicuous?"

"That's your all-or-nothing approach to life. If you can't walk in on your own two feet in high heels, stand around chatting all evening, and be the last to leave, you think you can't go at all. How about telling your hostesses ahead of time that you'll be there with your walker and will have to sit down to talk to people and tell them you'd like them to know that if you leave early, it's only because you need to go home and rest?" Dr. Hester suggested.

His suggestions made sense but I didn't follow them. I couldn't get up enough courage to face the people from my active days and be seen as a handicapped person, even if only temporarily handicapped. I stayed at home, lonely and angry at myself for allowing useless pride to keep me away from those stimulating people, ideas, and events.

Will I ever learn humility, I wondered, and put aside my concern about what other people think of me? Those people aren't my friends because of what I wear anyway. I'm going to have to face up to what my situation really is and go on out into the world, or withdraw from society, and that would be intolerable.

It was hard for me to let friends see me with a handicap, but for some reason it wasn't nearly as hard with a stranger. I was actually becoming a little flippant about it. One day, walking with the walker, I happened to reach the revolving door to a business at the same moment as a man walking with crutches and wearing a cast from his toes to his hip. He looked at me with my walker, I looked at him with his cast and crutches, and we both looked hopelessly at the spinning door. Shrugging my shoulders, I said, "Why don't we put us both together and get one good one?"

He laughed, I laughed, and we left to find a wider door.

It was time for another thirty-day checkup with Dr. Schultz. I was going into the fourth month since surgery and I wanted him to tell me I could stop using the walker, begin swimming, and start some tummy-tightening exercises. My hopes were high.

At the clinic Dr. Hurley, the orthopedic surgeon who'd assisted with so many of my operations, saw me come in and he hurried up the hall to say hello and ask how I was. "You're a strong one," he said in regard to the anterior spinal fusion.

Surprised and thinking of the trouble I had been, I said, "I don't feel like it. I feel like I've been a baby."

"No," he said consolingly. "This one was the big one."

In the examining room Dr. Schultz asked questions about my progress and observed my gait as he directed me to walk around the room. There was a pronounced lurch, as though I had a crippled leg. He told me to stand on one foot and hold my balance and do the same with the other foot. My left leg bore weight fine but my right leg collapsed from weakness the moment I put my full weight on it.

Regardless, I asked, "Can I stop using the walker now and just use the walls and furniture for balance?"

"No, you can't. What you will do over the next two or three months is gradually change to using a cane. When you're at home you can balance yourself by holding on to furniture, but whenever you leave your house you must use the walker or the cane."

He went on to explain, "We moved and cut a lot of your muscles and you were in bed long enough that you've lost strength in your muscles and they aren't strong enough to keep your leg from collapsing. The weakness also causes you to favor your stronger side and walk with that lurch I see. That pushes and pulls on your spinal fusion and puts too much stress on it. I don't want you to do that."

"Is it all right if I start swimming again?" I asked hopefully.

"No, but *if* the next X rays in thirty days look good and *if* your plugs are still in the holes in your spine, I'll let you begin walking in shallow water."

"Are you serious in saying the plugs can slip out?" I asked, appalled.

"Yes, they can pop right out of the holes," he answered.

"Well then, what kind of exercises can I do?" I asked. "Anything?"

"Yes, I want you to work on the muscles in your legs and hips. I want you to lie on your side on the floor, point your toes straight ahead, and raise your leg toward the ceiling. Work up to doing that five times a day and later work up to ten. Stop before you hurt or get tired, though."

"That's going to be easy," I bragged. "I can do a ninety-degree leg raise as many times as you want!"

My final question was, "What's my future in regard to wearing dress shoes with heels?"

Dr. Schultz replied, "*If* we get a good fusion, there's no reason why you can't wear what you want to someday."

At least one answer was what I wanted to hear, but I went home disappointed anyway. Dr. Schultz had cautioned me all along that an anterior spinal fusion is a hard one to get over and takes longer than the others, and he'd told me more than once that there was no guarantee that the operation would even be successful. Now it was all sinking in.

Deep in my soul I was already secretly afraid, because of the way my back felt, that there was still a problem with my spine, but I hadn't shared my fear with anyone because I didn't want to appear to be overly self-centered or an alarmist. Compared with other surgeries, it seemed that the level of pain was remaining too high for too long, I was tiring too fast, and there was increasing numbness in my foot, which caused me to stumble and trip when I walked or when I came down the stairs. It was difficult for me to cope with the uneasiness. I kept thinking I ought to be better by now and I should be working already.

My spirits needed a boost and I needed a success of some

kind so I decided to do the leg raises that had been so easy all my life. I usually had done fifty at a time, so it shouldn't be any problem to do half that number, even after surgery, I reasoned. I went upstairs and lay down on my side on the bedroom carpet. I tightened my muscles and exerted my strength to raise my right leg, but nothing happened. My leg didn't lift no matter how hard I strained to raise it.

I looked at my leg, tensed it, and tried again to raise it toward the ceiling. It took all the strength I could gather to lift it only four inches and I could only do that twice before my hip hurt too much to try again. The muscle strength simply was not there.

I could hardly believe what I was seeing and couldn't accept the fact that my strength had sunk so low. Maybe, I conceded to myself, maybe this operation really was the big one.

Chapter 17

SANTA FE

"Exercises must be as much a part of your daily life as brushing your teeth," Dr. Schultz said. "I want you to try these exercises I'm going to show you, but don't do anything that hurts you and stop before you get tired."

My resolve to become strong and healthy was renewed and I increased the number of exercises I did each day. I walked up and down the stairs ten times a day, a total of 260 steps, to strengthen my legs and I joined a health club in order to use their exercise equipment and eventually the swimming pool. It was slow work to regain my strength. For a few weeks I eased myself into the new exercises gradually, testing to find out what I could already do and what I would have to work up to.

Any one activity such as sitting still, standing, walking, or even lying down for a prolonged period of time still was extremely painful and Dr. Hester suggested techniques that I could use for the rest of my life to make myself regulate what I was doing. I learned to use a clock timer to remind myself to stop doing whatever it was I was engrossed in, move around, loosen up, and change activities. I purposely placed my glass of water in the next room when I was working at the desk so that I had to get up in order to get a drink. I ignored the nearest telephone when it rang and I walked to the phone in the next room to answer it. When I watched television I used the commercial breaks to do exercises. The techniques helped and my old habit of sticking to one job till I finished it, no matter how long it took, faded into the past.

Every day I went someplace in the car just for the joy of being out and active, and the bonus was that when I drove, my back didn't hurt as much. Does anyone need a taxi driver? I wondered. I might apply.

Then in late summer something came up that turned out to be a test of how far I had progressed and a reward for that progress. My insurance companies finally began to pay benefits after months of my paying the bills myself. There was one company, however, that denied any responsibility. Their home office and I exchanged notices, letters, phone calls, and documents, and we still couldn't reach a resolution. I telephoned the state insurance commissioner and talked with him about the problem, but it was of a nature that needed to be discussed in person with all of the documents in hand. The commissioner's office was at the State Capitol in Santa Fe, sixty miles north of Albuquerque.

How am I going to handle this? I asked myself. I don't want to ask any of my working friends to leave work for a day and drive me, nor do I want to disrupt the activities of my retired friends. Can I drive to Santa Fe myself? I'll have to use the walker, and the ancient, historic sidewalks in Santa Fe are rough to walk on. I can't walk very far and it's difficult to find a parking place near the plaza downtown. Can I make this trip by myself with no help from anyone?

I carefully considered everything I could do to guarantee, insofar as possible, that nothing would go wrong if I went alone. My car was new, the gas tank was full, and there was a handicap license plate on the back. The commissioner's office was in a government building, so the building was sure to have at least a few reserved spaces for handicap parking and easy access to the building. It would take less than a day to drive to Santa Fe, take care of my business, and get home again.

I told Stanford what I had in mind and he offered to drive me, but he didn't press me when I thanked him and said no. He understood my need to meet this challenge by myself.

I phoned the commissioner and made an appointment for the next day.

On the day of the trip Stanford and I ate breakfast together, and when he left for work, I put my insurance file and walker into the car and settled myself to drive. My back felt better already. I was so excited about the chance to handle my own affairs that I found myself grinning, giggling, and singing to the radio. It almost felt like the real me again. I didn't care that I probably looked silly. I was on my way to Santa Fe!

As I drove north on the freeway the hills and arroyos were green from summer rains and the sun was brilliant in a pure blue sky. Fluffy white cumulus clouds floated high above the Sangre de Cristo Mountains, the Sandias, and the Jemez. Volcanoes across the river valley were shades of purple and black above blue-gray cliffs and red hills. I reveled in the beauty all around me.

When I reached Santa Fe, I noticed the little river in the middle of town was swollen from the night's rain. Rushing water splashed and sparkled around and over the boulders and grassy banks. The plaza was washed clean and the Indian vendors sat in front of the Palace of the Governors and displayed their silver, gold, turquoise, coral, and shell jewelry on brightly striped blankets spread over the flagstone walk.

Geraniums and petunias were brilliant in the red clay pots and baskets hanging outside the hotels and shops. The outdoor cafes along the river sported blue and white umbrellas over tables where businessmen and tourists talked over hot, exotic coffee and croissants. Pine and pinion trees and the yuccas, chollas, and chamisas of the high desert still held droplets of rain that twinkled in the clear, bright sunlight. How can anyone bear to be sick and away from this? I wondered. How can I?

It was easy to find the state building where the insurance commissioner was housed and there was one parking space still open. I parked the car, picked up my file, unloaded the walker, and walked purposefully to the entrance. I was becoming tired and there was still the lobby to cross, the elevator to take to the third floor, and a long, long corridor ahead. By the time I reached the commissioner's office and was offered a chair, I was too exhausted to take another step.

We reviewed my documents, studied the performance rating

book for insurance companies, and considered the options for resolving the conflict. In short, the commissioner said he would be happy to file a complaint against the insurance company, but the fact of the matter was that the company was so big and I was so little that it probably wouldn't do me any good. It would most likely cost me additional time and expense and I'd still lose the $6,000 in question. I took the form required for filing the complaint but decided to talk with Stanford before I made a decision.

After the conference I went back down to my car and drove a few blocks to the Bull Ring, a restaurant I especially liked, and found their small parking lot hidden behind high adobe walls and clumps of burgundy hollyhocks. Hungry, I went into the charming adobe restaurant with the thick walls and woven rugs and was seated in the sunny patio, where flowers bloomed everywhere. The restaurant was the traditional watering hole for politicos and news people. Everyone seemed to know everyone else and talked table to table across the patio.

I sat in the sunshine, ate a small lunch, and listened to the conversations all around me. I savored the great pleasure of being there. When I left, I said good-bye to a few people who had said hello to me earlier. We didn't know each other, but in Santa Fe people are like that: friendly.

The drive home was one of joy. This day was a significant bench mark in my progress, the biggest challenge and the greatest success I'd had. Although I went to bed at three o'clock in the afternoon, exhausted and hurting, I was happier than I'd been for a long, long time.

The walker was unhandy and I wanted to be rid of it. I used it less and less at home and hated it more and more away from home. I felt as though I was ready to begin using a cane instead, so I got out the one I had wrapped with sterling silver and studded with turquoise gemstones as a gift for my father. After he was killed, my mother gave it back to me. It had sentimental value and I began to use it instead of the walker whenever I left home.

It was such a habit to take the walker that now, without it, I kept forgetting that I was supposed to take the cane. Stanford would come to take me out and time after time I'd pick up my purse, turn on the burglar alarm, lock the house, and be out the gate before I remembered the cane.

"Oh, nuts! I forgot my cane again! I'm sorry. I'll have to go back," I said one more time.

"I've got an idea," Stanford said as we unlocked the house, turned off the alarm, and picked up the cane. "Have you ever seen those chains people wear around their necks to keep track of their glasses? That's what I'm going to buy for you so you can chain your cane around your neck." He wasn't angry or impatient, but I got the message anyway.

For several summers Stanford and I had fun going to the mountains for Sunday breakfast cookouts. We took bacon and eggs, spiced, shredded potatoes and English muffins, and a percolator and cooked beside the stream at La Cienega. The pine trees were dewy and pale aspens shimmered in the morning breeze. Squirrels and blue jays chattered as they hopped around our table. The blazing fire smelled of pinion and cedar and the silence of the forest was peaceful.

This summer after the successful trip to Santa Fe, Stanford asked, "Do you think you feel good enough to go on a cookout? If you do and if you want to go, I'll buy the groceries and pack the equipment and I'll take care of the fire and do the cooking. I'll clean everything up and put it away when we get back. How's that for an offer?"

"That's the world's greatest offer and I accept!" I exclaimed excitedly. It would be terrific to be in the mountains again, especially to do something that Stanford liked as much as I did.

Early on Sunday morning Stanford packed everything into his station wagon and we drove up the canyon through the mountains and up the valley north to our turnoff. We talked all the way about how good the food was going to taste and how heavenly the perked coffee was going to smell. Then, as we came around a bend in the highway, we found the road blocked by sheriff's cars. Sheriff's deputies stood behind them, rifles laid across the roofs, pointed at us.

"Are we having fun yet?" Stanford cracked as he braked to a stop and the deputies surrounded us and peered into the car.

"We just want to check you and your car," the sheriff said as

Stanford presented his driver's license. "Last night there were seven inmates who escaped from the penitentiary this side of Santa Fe. They're all lifers and they're desperate. They've killed before and they don't give a damn about anybody. They need food, clothes, and money, and we think they came this way."

He waved his hand at the numbers of mountain ridges and canyons where the men could be and said, "There are homes and picnic areas all through these mountains. We're not forbidding you to go in there, but if you do, keep your eyes out for those guys and get out fast if you think you see them. We'll be here till we find them, so let us know if you see anyone who looks suspicious."

"What do you want to do?" Stanford asked me. "Our picnic area is right around the bend in a clearing that's in full view of the road."

"It's so close to the sheriff and his men and we can see all around us so well that if you feel all right about it, let's go ahead and have our cookout," I replied.

"Fine. We'll go on in but keep our eyes open."

We drove around the bend to the beautiful setting we had been looking forward to seeing again for our first cookout of the year, parked the car, and got out to smell the sweet, crisp mountain air.

"Wait!" Stanford suddenly whispered harshly and pointed to the steel trash container on the far side of the stream. "There's a man behind the dumpster digging through the trash."

The unshaved man, dressed in ragged, dirty clothes, suddenly saw us and jumped, startled. For a moment no one moved or spoke. Then the man pulled his arms and shoulders out of the dumpster, waved to us, and shouted, "Good morning! I don't wanna alarm ya, but there's some guys from the state pen runnin' around in these mountains and you'd better keep your eyes open for 'em." He began walking toward us. "I'm collectin' aluminum cans from all the picnic grounds. My civic group sells 'em and uses the money to send handicapped children to summer camp. Last year we collected enough cans to send nine children to camp and we think we can send twelve this year. Have ya got any cans ya wanna get rid of?"

We laughed in relief, wished him great success, and took our ice chest and picnic supplies out of the car. The incident was funny, but it might not have been. The escapees weren't caught until they had left a trail of terror, kidnapping, and rape through New Mexico, Arizona, and California.

This was one more experience with Stanford that told me the kind of man he was. I liked what I saw.

Chapter 18

TWO STEPS FORWARD
AND ONE STEP BACK

There were two big recent successes: Santa Fe and La Cienega. Now full of confidence, I was ready for another test, one that was more mundane but still necessary if I were to regain a normal way of life.

"I need to be able to buy groceries for myself and not have to ask Sarb Sarang to do it," I said to Stanford the next Saturday. "I'd like to see the fancy new supermarket that just opened and buy groceries there. Would you like to go with me and see it too?"

"Sure," he replied enthusiastically. "That company is going to build a store on one of my properties right away and I'd like to see what they're doing with this one."

I picked up my grocery list and cane and we drove to the store. At the front entrance there were electric carts with baskets and passenger seats built onto them so that a customer could ride around the store choosing his groceries and carrying them in the basket. "What a terrific idea for anyone who's old or disabled!" I exclaimed.

"You're not old, but do you want to ride on one?" Stanford asked, moving to turn one around for me.

"No, that's not for me. I don't want to look old or disabled. Let somebody who needs it use it."

We took a conventional grocery cart and began to explore the store and shop for the items on the list. The more aisles we walked, the worse my back and hip hurt. I didn't want to spoil our good time and I tried to keep going, but the pain became so excruciating and the fatigue so debilitating that I couldn't keep from crying.

Finally I said miserably, "I can't go on. Will you help me get to the deli section? There are some tables and chairs there where I can sit down for a few minutes."

People looked at the tears on my face and saw me try to drag my bad leg. I was embarrassed for Stanford and humiliated for myself. He didn't act dismayed at all, though. He patiently assisted me to a chair, finished the shopping, and went through the check-out while I rested.

The excursion was a failure. I was crushed. I should be able to buy my own groceries by now, I scolded myself, but instead I'm leaving the store in tears and going home to bed at one in the afternoon. I was distressed and depressed. What's the good of having those two successes if I can't have the one that I need the most?

I lay in bed during the afternoon and tried to work out some kind of system that would help me judge better whether or not my body was ready to succeed at a task. There had to be a better way to test myself and move ahead to the next challenge without any more setbacks like this one.

I asked Stanford what he thought about it.

"Is that your all-or-nothing syndrome? If you don't shop the entire store, are you such a failure that you're going to stay at home? Why not go back to a smaller store, take a grocery list, and do it more often instead of trying to do it all at once?"

His suggestions were sensible and calming. I would work on them.

A month had passed since Dr. Schultz had denied my requests to stop using the walker, do tummy exercises, and swim, and now it was time for a new examination and a new chance to ask to do the things I wanted to do.

"How are you feeling?" he asked before he began his examination and X rays.

I told him my back and hip still hurt too much to walk enough to shop, they troubled me to sit and stand, and I couldn't sleep well because they hurt too much. He directed me to stand up and balance on one foot and then the other, and told me to walk across the room and back with the cane and then without it. There was still a serious lurch in my gait and a twist in my fanny. He watched me critically, then, always the orthopedist, said disgustedly, "That may be sexy, but your back's not supposed to work like that. I'm going to take you to the physical therapist and have her evaluate your gait. She can design a program of physical therapy that will strengthen your back, hips, and legs and allow you to walk less painfully. You're still favoring your right side and placing stress on your spinal fusion. I don't want that!" He paused and put his hand on my shoulder. "I don't care how long it takes if we can just get you to hurting less, feeling better, and walking naturally."

Jo Ann, the physical therapist who had helped me so many times before, made an evaluation of my gait and muscle strength and explained her conclusions about the areas of greatest weakness. She demonstrated the exercises that would strengthen them. "For these inner thigh muscles, I want you to place something big and round and soft between your legs and squeeze them together. Start with five squeezes and work up to twenty."

Somehow that struck me as really funny, and laughing, thinking of other things, I said, "Couldn't I just make love a lot?"

"No," Jo Ann answered in her customary professional tone. "Those are your pelvic tilt muscles."

Respectful again, I took my list of exercises and stopped at a store on the way home to buy a big, soft ball, but I kept breaking out laughing all over again.

Dr. Hester increased his insistence on my breaking my old habits of pushing myself too hard. The rewards for successes had always been quick and the instant gratification fed my appetite to achieve even more, but now I was paying a heavy price in stress and pain.

"I'd like to measure the amount of tension in your back," Dr. Hester said during a session. "We have a biofeedback machine which will measure the amount of tension in your body and therefore measure the level of pain in different areas of your back when lying down, sitting, or standing."

"Why do you want to do that?" I asked.

"There are times when you look tense to me," he answered.

"I'm not tense. I used to be tense, but since I've been coming to you I'm so relaxed I feel like an amoeba," I defended myself. "My blood pressure has even dropped thirty-five points."

"Let me challenge you. You say you're relaxed. I believe you're tense. Let's take a reading and find out who's right."

"If we do it and you win the challenge and it shows I still do have too much tension, what can you do about it? I'm already practicing everything you've taught me about reducing tension."

"We can teach you to use biofeedback to zero in on specific areas of tension and pain and we can teach you how to control it just like biofeedback can be used to lower a person's blood pressure and heartbeat," he explained.

"All right, I'll do it, but just to humor you. I know how relaxed I am these days."

We scheduled the test with his associate.

"This is the biofeedback machine," she explained. "This meter registers the amount of tension which these electric leads pick up from certain locations on your back. I'll ask you to lie down on your tummy first and I'll attach the leads to two spots on your upper back, then two near your waistline, and finally two on your lower back." She continued to demonstrate the machine.

"Next, I'll ask you to sit up while I take the measurements in the same locations, and finally, I'll take a reading of those same places when you're standing. I'll be able to tell from the readings which areas and which positions cause you the greatest amount of stress and pain and those readings will be the basis for your training to use the biofeedback machine to relieve tension and pain. Do you have any questions before we begin?"

I didn't, so she started the test. I felt thoroughly relaxed and from time to time I was able to see the meter and read the needle bouncing in a low range. I'm going to win the challenge, I thought. This machine proves that I'm not tense, just as I said.

The diagnostician finished the test, wrote her report, walked me to Dr. Hester's office, and handed the report to him. He studied it without any comment.

"How did I do?" I asked cockily, anticipating his surrender.

"You averaged six to eight points on the scale in most areas."

That didn't tell me anything. "What's the range?" I asked, still waiting for him to give in.

"The ordinary person on a bad day would score two to three points," he answered. "You scored far above normal."

"How can that be? I'm not tense or stressed anymore and I don't rush around doing a million things all at once like I always used to do. All I ever do nowadays is relax!"

"If we had tried to measure you six months ago when you were running a business with a broken spinal fusion, you would have been so far above the top of the meter that we couldn't have gotten a reading on you," he explained. "You don't even know how a normal person is supposed to feel. We can help you teach yourself to reduce your tension and pain to a normal level, however."

"Instead of starting biofeedback training can't I just work on my own to try to bring down the level of tension? I've taken training from some of the best people in the country and I've taught relaxation techniques to others, so I ought to be able to help myself do it."

"Sure, you can do that," he said. "Use all the techniques you have, and later if you want to learn biofeedback, we can start you on it. We can always hope."

"I'm living on *esperanza* anyway," I offered. "Hope is the best thing I have: Hope that I'll get well, hope that I can go to work, hope that my back problems are over. I'll work on the relaxation techniques and hope that they help."

In addition to increasing the amount of time I spent in relaxation activities, I also increased other activities. Dr. Hester taught me to keep my mind active as a distraction from the pain and during the autumn months, I completed writing a collection of poetry about the sea, matched the poetry with photographs I had taken, and recorded a reading of the verses with a background of beautiful music. I sent a selection of the poems to various publishers and they were accepted for publication in their anthologies. It was fun and exciting and it gave me a warm feeling of accomplishment—of success at having health good enough to finish something I started.

I was also writing nonfiction articles for magazines, so I made a series of appointments to interview artists and business people and wrote profiles of them. One of the interviews was with Dirk and Jan Schneider, artists whose paintings are shown all around the world. As we sat at lunch in their art gallery, they asked about my back and what problems it had caused. I talked about some of the problems and, feeling as though I knew them well enough to confide it, I said, "It's really hard to maintain a healthy romantic relationship, though, when you're always flat on your back in bed."

Without a second's hesitation Dirk said, looking innocent, "I always thought that was the best way!"

Jan and I, at first shocked to hear such a remark from staid Dirk, collapsed in laughter.

All these months I speculated about what kind of work I'd be able to do and I read everything I could find about occupations to look into. It looked as though it would be important for me to know how to use a word processor, so I bought one, had it installed, and began to teach myself to use it. I had trouble learning all the functions and asked Stanford to help me since he had one in his office. He sat down at the desk and worked diligently for an hour while I silently watched, but he was unable to make my word processor respond to his commands.

Abruptly he turned off the switch, stood up, and said with disgust, "I can't make it work. I was a genius till I was six, but after that I outgrew it."

Cracking up, I was on my own again.

I became able to do more of my housework, but I left the difficult tasks for Sarb Sarang. I was able to do all of my own grocery shopping and errands and I met friends sometimes for lunch. I kept doing my exercises and I was stronger but not at all well. My back and hip hurt badly, and there was a spot on the outer point of my hipbone that was too tender to touch or to lie on. Also my thigh from my knee up burned, felt irritated and agitated, and hurt so much that I couldn't stand any but the softest fabrics to touch it.

Dr. Schultz, concerned, sent me to Dr. Mora for another neurological examination.

"There are several possible causes for both of these problems," he began, "but I don't recommend any more surgery. That might not help you and it could make you worse. You can try to live with it and eventually it will wear off or I can inject anesthetic into those nerves and take some of the pain out right away. Some ultrasound treatments might help you, too, and I'll talk to Dr. Schultz about giving you some."

I agreed to the ultrasound and asked for the injections to help me also. Dr. Mora gave me a series of five injections into the nerves over a period of several weeks, but they didn't give me enough relief from the pain and he discontinued them. Jo Ann, the physical therapist, gave me the ultrasound treatments, but the improvement after a month of the treatments was negligible, so they too were discontinued.

Dr. Mora was right in predicting that the hypersensitivity in my thigh would diminish over time and I was grateful for that. Then, suddenly and without warning, all of the sensitivity and more returned to my thigh.

I took a shower and went to bed about eleven o'clock one night, somewhat aware that my thigh hurt more than it had for a while. I wondered why. At two in the morning there was searing pain in my thigh, my nerves were so agitated they made me feel nervous and explosive, and every twenty or thirty seconds a jolt like electricity zapped my leg so hard that it bounced it off the bed. I got up and walked the floor for the rest of the night, careful that no clothing touched my fiery, itching, hurting thigh.

At daylight, so tired I could hardly stand up, I looked carefully at my thigh. It was a patch of redness, hot and feverish to the touch with a dime-sized blister in the center. An hour later there were three more blisters.

At 8:30 A.M. I phoned Dr. Mitchell's receptionist. "I probably need to see a doctor today. Could Dr. Mitchell or any of the others see me on short notice?"

"Lucy, I'm sorry but Dr. Mitchell is the only doctor in the office this week. The others are off for the holidays. Can you tell me why you need him?" she asked.

"Sure. There are two problems. I think I have poison ivy, even though I can't imagine where I got it, and it's on top of the thigh where I already have the trouble with the nerve damage. The other problem is that I've had constant vaginal bleeding for four months and the medications that Dr. Mitchell gave me haven't been helping. I don't feel good."

"Can you be here in twenty minutes? Our family nurse practitioner can see you and if she needs Dr. Mitchell, she'll get him," she replied.

Genara Griego, the family nurse practitioner, took me to her examining room. "Let's look at your leg first," she said. She examined the feverish redness and the blisters and said, "You have shingles."

"What's shingles?" I asked. "It looks like poison ivy."

"Shingles, or herpes zoster, is a painful virus in the nerve. It's related to chicken pox and anyone who's ever had chicken pox has the virus in his system for the rest of his life. It can surface when certain conditions weaken the body's defenses," Mrs. Griego explained.

"How do I get rid of it? It's driving me crazy!"

"Unfortunately," she said, "there's not any good cure for shingles, just like there's no good cure for other viruses. I could give you a prescription for painkillers, but you'd just react to them and feel even worse. I will give you a cortisone ointment to rub on the area in its present stage and an ointment that has silver in it to rub on the blisters when they break to keep them from scarring your leg. I'm afraid you're just going to be miserable until the virus runs its course, probably a couple of weeks. I'm really sorry that I can't do very much for you."

I covered my leg as she asked, "Now what's this about bleeding? Your chart shows that Dr. Mitchell has made several changes in your medications to try to cycle you. Didn't they help?"

"No, not yet. The bleeding started four months ago and hasn't stopped. Dr. Mitchell said he'd try to get my system balanced, but if he couldn't I'd need to see a gynecologist and have a D&C. I told him I didn't want any more surgery, even minor surgery, but now I don't know what to do," I said.

Mrs. Griego reviewed my medications and consulted with Dr. Mitchell.

"Here's what we're going to do. But if you're not stopped in another two months, you will need that D&C," she said and explained what pills and shots she was going to give me.

I went home, lay down on the bed, and thought about how uneven the healing process is—one day good and one day bad—and contemplated the virtues of acceptance, tolerance, and patience that I didn't seem to have enough of. How did other people develop them? I wondered. How will I ever have enough to manage these constant illnesses and cope with my back too? I keep living on *esperanza* . . . hope . . . but I feel as though it's running out.

"It's hard to keep from getting discouraged," I confided to Stanford at breakfast after a painful, sleepless night. "What I need is a support group of people who have similar problems and have had the same kinds of medical experiences and can share what they've learned about coping. There must be an easier way to learn what to do than the way I'm doing it, one bad experience at a time."

"Why don't you start a group yourself?" he asked. "You're a counselor with plenty of experience leading discussion groups."

It was a good idea that I liked, but I didn't yet trust myself to always feel good enough to do the regular planning that would be needed for each session or to have the energy to conduct the discussions. That was an idea that would have to wait.

Chapter 19

I DON'T KNOW
WHAT ELSE WE CAN DO

It was time once again for a follow-up exam with Dr. Schultz. "It's been over nine months since the last operation and I still feel so bad that there must be something wrong in my back. There's sharp pain when I move, the pain stabs me if I twist, and my back aches too much to stand up even long enough to buy stamps at the post office. Something deep in the back of my hip makes walking so difficult that I only get halfway through the drugstore, and have to drag this leg forward with each step. I have to go to the grocery store twice as often as I normally would because I can't walk all the way through it at any one time. I hardly go anyplace else or do anything more than what I have to do. I do my exercises and I rest but I can't sleep at night because of pain. What can be causing it?" I asked Dr. Schultz before he started his examination.

Dr. Schultz looked at me thoughtfully. "You'll be better off when you accept the fact that you're going to continue to have problems and that you can't ever do some of the things you used to do. There are some problems you're just going to have to live with. You can go on hoping that things will get better and you can do a lot to maintain your health and perhaps improve it, but you'll still have to keep coping."

Sympathetically and apologetically he continued, "I would do anything to help you get rid of your health problems and make you feel good, but I don't know what else to do. We've done multiple operations on you, we've given you all kinds of physical therapy and treatments, you've been through exercise and swimming programs, and we've given injections into your spine and injections into your hip. We're about to run out of things to do with you. The fact of the matter is you frustrate the hell out of me." He was angry. Then sheepishly he added, "I shouldn't talk to you that way, should I? You're a nice lady."

"Dr. Schultz," I replied, "you and I have been together for so many years and been through so many bad times that you've seen me at my very worst. There's nothing you could say that would offend me."

"All right," he said, making another start, "suppose there is something wrong that isn't showing up on any of the tests or X rays you've had. Suppose the increased pain is not associated with the shingles—many times it is—and suppose your uric acid level is normal and your gout is not causing the pain. There's only one more test we can do that will show us if there's some problem we're missing. That's the MRI. If we give it to you and we find something wrong, I don't know what we can do about it. I won't do another operation on you! Each back operation lowers your chances of being helped. If we did go into your back and were as gentle and careful with your nerves as we could possibly be, we could still cause enough damage that you could get your foot drop again and I don't know what the chances are for making a second comeback."

Choosing my words carefully I said, "I've gone for months trying everything you've suggested that might help and hoping for improvement, but I just keep getting worse. I don't know what's wrong or if it can be fixed. I don't know what's in my future or what I'll have to cope with. I don't even know whether or not I'll be able to work. It's hard for me to stay optimistic when I can't see any light at the end of the tunnel. I'm about to get a discouragement problem."

Dr. Schultz sighed. "I want Dr. Mora to examine you again and let me know if he has any more ideas. If he thinks we should do the MRI, we'll do it."

"What is that?" I asked, unfamiliar with the term.

"MRI means Magnetic Resonance Imaging and you might say

that it's a sophisticated form of CT scan. It'll pick up anything that's there to see. The CT scan is done with X rays, but the MRI is a magnetic-field type of image and you don't get any radiation. The pictures are very exact and anatomical and are in gradation of white, gray, and black." He pulled several negatives of MRI pictures out of a manila envelope, hung them on his viewing glass, and pointed out various features of bone, nerve, and muscle.

"A person who is trained to read these pictures can pick up any problem that exists."

"How do you take the test?" I asked.

"There's a magnetic imaging center down the street: that new building in the medical complex. Patients are referred by their doctor for the test and it costs about nine hundred dollars. They set an appointment for you and when you get there they show you a video tape explaining the procedure for using the two-and-a-half-million-dollar machine. They'll have you change into a gown, but they won't give you any shots. They'll have you lie down on a specially padded table and slip you into the machine. You'll feel like you're inside a thermos bottle and if you have any trouble with claustrophobia, you won't be able to take the test. The photographs are made through the use of powerful magnetic forces, radio waves, and supercomputers. While pictures are being made, you'll hear clicking and clanking sounds. All you have to do is lie perfectly still. If we send you to have the test done, you'll be there about an hour and a half or so."

Thinking back to the very beginning of my back problems, I wanted to know why I was here and asked, "Why did I ever have all these back problems in the first place?"

"Your discs degenerated," Dr. Schultz began. "That's a common occurrence and we know from studying cadavers that degeneration begins during youth and the amount of degeneration varies from one person to another. One factor is arthritis. Another is simple wear and tear. It can be a result of both of them or of other things. Some people seem more disposed to having those problems than others, but why it affected you in the way it did we just don't know."

I made an appointment to see Dr. Mora and explained to him why Dr. Schultz wanted him to reevaluate me.

After the examination, Dr. Mora said, "I don't know what's

causing your problems and I don't know what I can do about it even if I find out. I will not operate on you again! There comes a time when surgery makes things worse, not better."

"Do you have any ideas for Dr. Schultz or me?" I asked.

"No, I don't know what else to do for you. You might try the TENS again and you might have an MRI study done. I'll talk to Dr. Schultz about it, but I think you're just going to have to live with what you have."

Is this the last resort? I wondered. Doesn't medical science have anything else for me? Is there nothing that will cure me or at least keep me from becoming worse? What will my future be and do I have the character to cope with the possibilities that are looking more and more like probabilities? I'll wait to find out what the doctors decide to do. If I take an MRI, it might show nothing more than these old problems that still aren't well. On the other hand, it might show some new thing that's wrong, but no one knows of anything that can be done about it.

I drove home low on hope, but stubborn and still resolved to try to cope with what I had and think about how I could do it—even if just for one step at a time, starting now.

Chapter 20

DEAR ABBY

Several years ago Abigail Van Buren, known throughout the world as Dear Abby, flew into Albuquerque to address a large convention of journalists. She and her entourage left the plane and as they entered the airline waiting room, the waiting crowd parted to make a path. I was standing in the front row. Abby, passing through the crowd, saw me, walked directly to me, and said, to my amazement, "Beautiful!" Dumbfounded even to be noticed by her, let alone paid the compliment by such a lovely lady, I'll cherish that gracious compliment forever. Now, much later and with so many things changed in my life, Abby affected me in another way through her newspaper column of New Year's resolutions.

On New Year's Day Stanford and I sat in front of the fire and lingered over our morning coffee while we read the *Albuquerque Journal.* Abby's column caught my eye and, as I read her list of New Year's Resolutions, it seemed as though Abby had summarized everything the doctors, psychologist, Stanford, and my experiences had taught me during the past year. Abby phrased them into a creed a back patient can live by.

Every resolution struck a nerve and made me see quite clearly the mistakes I'd made. I always tried to overcome all my problems at once and Abby addressed that issue. I needed to improve my mind and be more interested and interesting. It was necessary that I do things that were positive for my health.

Pain often made me irritable, impatient, and sometimes tact-less. There were times when it was hard for me to be happy and agreeable. My experiences at relaxing were all new to me. I needed to take additional responsibility for myself. And so on down the page.

Abby's resolutions were so powerful that I obtained her per-mission to print them here. Maybe they'll fit you as they do me. Here is her column dated December 31, 1987:

Reader Benefits from Living Life
a Day at a Time*

DEAR ABBY: Last New Year's Eve you published some New Year's resolutions. I cut that column out and taped it on my bathroom mirror where I could read it every morn-ing. I want you to know that it has helped me to become a better person. I am not saying that I kept every one of those resolutions every day, but I kept most of them and they have now become habits that have made a remarkable improvement in my personality and character.

I hope you will run it every New Year's Eve. I'm sure it will benefit many others as it has me.—NEVER TOO OLD.

DEAR NEVER: My "resolutions" column has become an established annual tradition.

DEAR READERS: These New Year's resolutions are based on the original credo of Alcoholics Anonymous. I have taken the liberty of using that theme with some vari-ations of my own:

Just for today I will live through this day only and not set far-reaching goals to try to overcome all my problems at once. I know I can do something for 12 hours that would appall me if I felt that I had to keep it up for a lifetime.

Just for today I will be happy. Abraham Lincoln said, "Most folks are about as happy as they make up their minds to be." He was right. I will not dwell on thoughts that depress me. I will chase them out of my mind and replace them with happy thoughts.

Just for today I will adjust myself to what is. I will face reality. I will correct those things that I can correct and accept those things I cannot correct.

Just for today I will improve my mind. I will not be a

mental loafer. I will force myself to read something that requires effort, thought, and concentration.

Just for today I will do something positive to improve my health. If I'm a smoker, I'll make an honest effort to quit. If I'm overweight, I'll eat nothing I know is fattening. And I will force myself to exercise—even if it's only walking around the block or using the stairs instead of the elevator.

Just for today I will be totally honest. If someone asks me something I don't know, I will not bluff; I'll simply say, "I don't know."

Just for today I'll do something I've been putting off for a long time. I'll finally write that letter, make that phone call, clean that closet or straighten out those dresser drawers.

Just for today before I speak I will ask myself, "Is it true? Is it kind?" And if the answer to either of those questions is negative, I won't say it.

Just for today I will make a conscious effort to be agreeable. I will look as good as I can, dress becomingly, talk softly, act courteously, and not interrupt when someone else is talking. Just for today I'll not improve anybody except myself.

Just for today I will have a program. I may not follow it exactly, but I will have it thereby saving myself from two pests: hurry and indecision.

Just for today I will have a quiet half hour to relax alone. During this time I will reflect on my behavior and get a better perspective on my life.

Just for today I will be unafraid. I will gather the courage to do what is right and take the responsibility for my own actions. I will expect nothing from the world, but I will realize that as I give to the world, the world will give to me.

Have a happy, healthy New Year. And pray for peace!

LOVE, ABBY

P.S. If you are driving tonight, don't drink. And if you're drinking, please don't drive.

Chapter 21

COPING EMOTIONALLY

There is no problem, personal or technical,
that you can't solve.

D. A. Dobkins

Regardless of what the doctors were going to decide about having me take the MRI exam or not, my life was at another turning point. There weren't going to be any miracles to solve my problems. It had been so many years since I had awakened to a day without pain that I didn't remember what it was like to feel good and it was probably just as well that I didn't.

There was no value in cataloguing all the things that were wrong with my health and my back or in looking around me at all the people who were so terribly more ill or injured than I was. All that did was make me feel even worse that they were so sick and that I was helpless to do anything for them.

It looked to me as though the way for me to find some direction for my future was to look back at my past and see what I had learned and then intensify my efforts to practice those things that might help. On a legal pad labeled *Coping*, I drew four columns and sublabeled them *Emotionally, Physically, Socially,* and *Financially*. I began to list what I'd learned and I was surprised to find that the columns weren't big enough to hold it all.

That in itself pointed to one thing I'd learned: it helps if I keep my mind occupied. It isn't good for me to think about myself too much. I have a better attitude and outlook on life if I direct my thoughts to the people and activities that stimulate me. Friends, family, books, newspapers, journals, music, television, and getting out of the house do a lot to keep me interested in what's going on in the world and keep me distracted from my pain.

It's a great help for me to write, I learned, whether it's a letter, poetry, magazine articles, or this book, and to express to someone else what I see and how I feel about it. Whenever someone reads what I write and likes it, I get so excited that I can hardly contain myself. Especially important to me is being able to talk with other people and exchange knowledge, thoughts, and ideas. I need to be with people, not alone.

I find that I have a deeper need to nurture my relationships with my friends now than before and I have a better sense of the importance of sharing their lives right now. Life has too many twists and turns that can take someone away from me tomorrow. I used to put off phoning, writing, or visiting friends, because we were all so busy and I figured there would always be time later. Now I believe it's important to do the significant things today.

I learned, too, to be more open about myself. I no longer have to try to be so strong that I can solve all my own problems, be invincible, and be emotionally independent of other people. These times of illness have taught me the value of leaning on other people and drawing on their strength when I need to. It's finally okay not to be Superwoman.

Still difficult, but I'm learning, is how to compromise. It takes effort to settle for less than I used to. For instance, I can't be comfortable at a concert or basketball game or movie where I have to sit still and straight for a prescribed period of time, but I can enjoy performances at home with recordings, television, and video cassettes. I can't go dancing with my friends, but I can invite them over for dinner by the fire.

It's essential to my mental state, I know, to live in a clean and attractive home. Part of my therapy while recuperating from surgery was to get my new house finished, and while I was at home most of the time it was easy to schedule workmen. I drew the plans for a low-maintenance yard with redwood decking, potter's benches, a firewood box, and planters, and designed the landscaping. I hired contractors and nurserymen to do the work. Next I designed built-ins for the closets, vanities, cupboards, and storage rooms and had cabinetmakers build them.

Finally, the best fun of all, I asked Emily Zander, the interior designer for my homes for several years, to help me with this house. Emily had been in the same hospital that I was in and had a spinal fusion at the same time. Now she was working and doing fine. She came over to study the house, and we began to choose fabrics and furniture. By the time Emily finished she'd turned my house into a home filled with music and art, softness and sunlight, a lovely and comfortable place to get well in and stay well in.

It's emotionally fulfilling to me to visit my funny, delightful, dear mother. She still has a full social schedule and she goes to exercise class and a health lecture every morning. When talking about her class, however, she did say, "It does hurt a little to touch my head to my knees." What an inspiration she is for all of us!

Regularly, business associates come in to town and over lunch or dinner they keep me up-to-date on their business and personal lives. That helps me cope with being out of the mainstream of work. Someone I especially enjoy seeing when she comes into town is Lachmi Raichandani of Hong Kong. She is always sunny and happy and brings me up-to-date on news from her home: industry, the economy, the British government, and trends. We speculate on what life in Hong Kong will be like in 1997, when the British turn over control to the Chinese. Lachmi owns a high-rise condominium in downtown Hong Kong but comes to the United States and Canada to visit her family and friends and to do graduate work at the University of New Mexico. She did her university administration internship under my supervision a few months before I hurt my back at school and I was very impressed with her.

Later, after the store was established and running smoothly, my partner and I negotiated a lease to open a second store and we contracted with Peter Grivas to design the interior. Businessmen and brokers in other states asked us to franchise the store and let them buy in. We needed a pool of talented managers. Tom Wingfield was the first and Lachmi came to mind very quickly as a good additional manager. Unfortunately my back turned bad shortly afterwards and we had to scrap all of the plans.

For my best emotional health I find that I can't dwell on how much I miss the store and our customers. It's better if I don't think about it or talk about it or drive past it. That's a situation, one of a series, that I simply have to accept. To use Jeanne Scher's technique, I have to put it into a small black bag and fling it over my shoulder.

Part of my day-to-day plan, in addition to accepting the losses I don't have any control over, is to keep the stress out of my life. I try to focus on doing the things I am capable of doing at a pace my system can tolerate. If I can't be a greyhound winning the race, I'll try to be a turtle who's slower but steady enough to at least finish it.

I practice all of the relaxation techniques that Dr. Buscaglia and others taught me: tightening and relaxing muscles, breathing deeply, bringing to mind the memories of peaceful moments, and creating images of how I want to be. I have in my mind a happy image of my family and it gives me considerable pleasure. In my image I find a way to help other people cope with back problems; my beautiful, widowed sister finds someone she can love forever; my brother Dave becomes well off and famous for his patents in genetics and telemetry; my brother Jim wins his race to be a United States congressman from Colorado and we pick up our mother and Stanford and whisk them away for a big party in Washington, D.C.

Another thing that helps me cope is to set goals for myself, both short range and long range, and to plan rewards for success. Some of my favorite prizes are lunch with Stanford in Albuquerque's Old Town, a new book or recording, or an afternoon in Santa Fe.

Extremely vital to me is my relationship with Stanford. I want him to know every day that I treasure his friendship and that I have fun being with him. I used to try to hide my distress when my back was cranky and I felt rotten, but I don't believe that's the fair way to treat Stanford. A friend wants to be of help and can't really know how to help if you don't let him know what you need, whether it's a hug and hope, or a pain pill and a quiet nap.

Many of us were brought up to be stoic, to grit our teeth, lock our jaws, lift our chins, choke back any sobs, and carry on with our work. I don't believe in doing that anymore either. If you present an exterior that hides your true physical and emotional state, your friends have to base their responses on what they see. If what they see is the opposite of what you really feel, how can they do the things that will help you? If you hurt like the blazes but smile and insist you're fine, and if you really need some hot soup and a good sleep, are you going to be taken care of? Nope. You're going to be invited to go do something interesting, exciting, and exhausting.

I'm trying to learn to give out the right signals, honest signals, to the people around me and I'm trying to read theirs correctly, too. That doesn't mean, however, that I lay bare my soul or cry on every shoulder. I don't gripe about every ache and pain, even to my doctors, but I keep a private daily log and when a complaint lasts long enough that it becomes a pattern and doesn't improve, I go for help and I do complain.

Most of all I try to be optimistic and cheerful while I am learning to cope.

A University of Pittsburgh professor of psychiatry was quoted as saying, "If, when people confront difficulties in their lives, they believe the outcome will be good, they're more likely to obtain a good outcome than if they believe it will eventually be bad."

An optimistic person is one who concentrates on ways to solve problems, formulates plans for action and makes alternative plans in case something goes wrong, accepts that nothing can be done about the situation that turned out wrong, and moves ahead with his life.

I have cherished Stanford throughout the years, during good times and bad, and hoped that our relationship could someday become permanent. However, it seemed grossly unfair to foist upon him the frequent disruptions to our friendship due to problems with my health, especially my spine; and I certainly did not want to put him in a situation in which he would have any responsibility for my ongoing, enormous medical bills.

Now I see that he is not afraid of the disruptions. We are both learning to cope with them and are staying emotionally healthy. With my medical costs under control, I have one less worry. Our lives have settled into a more relaxed and optimistic mode, and we are finally able to turn our thoughts to planning an exciting future. Time's a-wastin'!

Chapter 22

COPING PHYSICALLY

Doctors, nurses, and physical therapists taught me practical ways to take better care of my health and I practice them conscientiously. One of the lessons that came from my good medical experiences with doctors is to choose the best doctors, establish a good rapport with them, provide them with enough accurate and detailed health information for them to make correct diagnoses, and then rely on their judgment. I'm very good at knowing when something is wrong with me, but I'm really bad at making the right diagnosis and determining my own treatment, like when I decided that what I needed was a hip transplant when there was nothing at all wrong with my hip.

I'm also learning to see a doctor earlier during an illness instead of waiting so long that it's an established and seriously hard-to-cure illness.

After the medical experiences I've had, I know that I need to follow the doctors' instructions, regardless of whether they make any sense to me or are boring. The doctors have been right so consistently that I have faith in what they tell me.

Part of the route to recovery and continued good health is a regular, daily exercise program. On the worst days, when the pain is too severe to even think of going to the health club, I still do isometric exercises and I walk up and down the stairs at home as one form of conditioning. Almost every day I do the exercises the doctors and physical therapists taught and several times a week I do go to the health club to use their exercise equipment and swimming pool.

I haven't tried acupuncture, acupressure, or massage yet, but I'm interested in learning about them.

One of the recommendations for back patients is that they limit their weight. I'm paying attention to the number of calories I burn and I'm watching my caloric intake. Stanford and I are both reading the newest publications about good nutrition and cholesterol and fat control. Now that I'm not working in a business where I'd dash out to a restaurant for a fast meal, I'm cooking at home and practicing new, healthier ways of cooking. I'm also avoiding caffeine most of the time, since caffeine can increase tension.

In addition to those practices I continue to use all of the relaxation techniques that were taught me in order to keep my stress level low and reduce the pain, which is exacerbated by stress. In a series of recordings of nature sounds called "Environments," by the Atlantic Recording Corporation, there is a cassette called *Seashore* that I enjoy by the hour. The sound of the surf relaxes me.

I don't want to seem immodest but it also relaxes me to read my own poetry or to play my poetry recorded with a background of music. There are two poems in particular that bring back memories of happy, sunny, family vacations on the coast of Mexico: "Hispanic Christmas" and "Winter Clam Beds."

HISPANIC CHRISTMAS

At Christmastime in Mexico
    In our village on the bay
Está tradición
    To honor our Lord this way.

Mis madre, padre, y hermanos
    Will walk to the church and pray
When the ruby flames of sunrise
    Change the sea from somber gray.

Todo el día, amigos and I
    Will build castles and swim and fish,
Chop oysters and mussels and dig for clams,
    And catch all the crabs we wish.

At nightfall a gentle ocean breeze,
  Our sweet guitars by the fire,
And the melody of an ebbing tide
  Will soothe like a heavenly choir.

Tall candles lit at the glowing flame
  Will guide our eager feet
In the Holy Procession from door to door
  Seeking the manger sweet.

We'll ask at each home, "Is there room at the inn?"
  "Lo siento, no está aquí."
But the door of the church will open wide;
  "Is the Christ Child here?" "Yes, *si.*"

We'll smile and kneel before the saints,
  Our hearts filled with joy from above.
We'll gaze upon the Jesus babe
  And worship in tender love.

WINTER CLAM BEDS

Across the strait beyond white surf,
  past dunes of sand and grass,
  in shallow brine lie clam beds
  warmed by hazy sun.

An emerald tropic jungle
  cuts the chill of northern winds
  and we hear the haunting calls
  of long-necked birds.

Our sun-browned children bring small spades
  but mostly dig with stubby hands
  in gritty, brown-gray mounds
  where tender clams can soon be found
  in this low tide.

Each rough, white clam shown 'round with smiles
  is offered to the child who has but few
  and little hands reach out to hold the prize.
  We ask, within which child resides the greater joy?

And then, too fast, the chilly ocean tide
  comes surging through our realm. So soon?

Must we stop digging clams so soon?
How fast the day has flown.

We watch in awe the red-rose evening sky
    tint jagged, purple, granite peaks,
    and flocks of egrets fly to hidden nests
    in limbs of darkened mangrove trees.

Weary, hungry, though content,
    we store our memories and drag our spades
    and pails of clams
    beside the foaming sea toward home.

There's a theory that severe stress can cause the brain to release large amounts of painkilling endorphins, the body's own substance, and also increase the ability to tolerate even more stress. The body learns to need increasing amounts of stress to trigger a greater output of endorphins to kill the pain caused by the stress it aimed to reduce in the first place.

My sister sent me a copy of an article called "Mind Over Disease" from the April 1987 *Reader's Digest,* in which one of the steps suggested for combating stress that can be damaging to your health is to accept what you can't control. If you have a condition that is going to stay with you forever, stop fighting it, change your focus, and work around it. I'm trying to do that.

It helps me control pain if I avoid doing the things that obviously aggravate back problems, such as vacuuming the carpet, moving anything heavy, lifting things, stooping down, leaning over, or reaching up. I try to arrange the cupboards and closets in such a way that the items I use the most often are at midlevel. If I absolutely must lift something, I bend my knees, not my back. I don't yank on doors that are heavy or push anything that's bulky or heavy, and I have a long-handled tong to reach and grasp items that are high.

Two of the most helpful innovations were Stanford's ideas. The first thing he did was jack up my queen-sized waterbed and place six-inch blocks under the legs. It is easier to sit down on it and get up, and it's much easier to change the linens. The second idea was to build a six-inch platform for the washer and dryer so I wouldn't have to lean over so far to use them.

Sarb Sarang does all of the hard housework and cleans the

windows, and when the yard needs heftier care than I can give it, I get help.

Dr. Hester taught me to pace myself and alternate my activities with rest. He made me conscious of fatigue and stress being linked together and I now discipline myself to stop whatever I'm doing before it becomes hurtful. I'm becoming skilled at taking a break from my desk and lying down when I need to, walking up and down the stairs a few times, doing some exercises, or working in the kitchen until my muscles loosen up and I feel more relaxed.

Dr. Schultz suggested that I go to the State Motor Vehicle Department and fill out a form to obtain a handicap license plate for the car. I did go to their office, was helped promptly, and had a minimum amount of standing in line. Dr. Schultz filled out his portion of the form and I mailed it with my two-dollar check to the capitol in Santa Fe. It took about a month to receive a metal handicap license plate. It would be extremely difficult for me to manage without it and I appreciate the privilege of having it when I need it.

Pacing myself, I plan my errands for the week in such a way that I don't fill any one day too full of activities that are physically taxing. For instance, on the day that I go to the post office, I don't go to the grocery store or drugstore.

After the last back operation, my back hurt too much to sleep on the waterbed I had so I bought a newer type that has a series of small, independent tubes of water which mold to fit the hollows and curves of a person's body and make sleeping more comfortable. It's a good design for me, yet I still can't sleep through a night because of the pain. I'm experimenting and I'm finding that I rest best if I sleep a short time at night and take a little nap or two during the day. It keeps my muscles and bones from settling in one position so long that they become stiff.

Another method for me to get relief from pain is to lie down on my back, bend my knees, and tuck a couple of pillows under them to lessen the amount of arch in my spine and the strain on my lower back. A heating pad helps relieve muscle spasms and it makes me feel terrific to be in a hot tub, sauna, or steam room. Always wherever I am I try to keep my back from becoming chilled and the muscles from becoming tense. Since it isn't helpful for me to take pain pills and there are times when the pain is too horrendous to stand, I work my way through this repertoire of pain-fighting techniques and try to get relief naturally.

It would be evasive of me if I didn't mention the value of good sex for a person's health and sense of well-being. Frankly, it's not always easy for a back patient to make love. To begin with, severe trauma and stress can cause the hormones in both men and women to diminish temporarily, lessening the libido until the patient regains his health and his body can restore its own normal levels of hormones, particularly testosterone in men and testosterone, progesterone, and estrogen in women. There's no need for the patient to be alarmed or upset, though. Patience, time, consultations with his or her physician, and a loving relationship do help return everything to normal.

Also, there are times when back pain and general fatigue rob the patient of interest and energy. That doesn't negate the need for affection and intimacy, however. You don't have to set off the smoke alarms every time you make love in order for it to be good. How cozy and tender it is to lie in the arms of some-one you love, touching, feeling, caressing, talking, laughing, and playing. In my bed I guess you might call it Lucy's Pil-lowtalk.

Another important aspect in coping with my health is to fol-low the program of medications, vitamins, and minerals that my endocrinologist worked out for me. I am on lifetime cortisone, and cortisone lowers a person's immunity to illness and makes it harder to get over illnesses and injuries, so I try to avoid high-risk situations that could easily cause an illness. I've had too many of them already, including paratyphoid, pneumonia, mononucleosis, epiglottitis, tuberculosis, bronchitis, and other illnesses, to be blasé or careless about my health.

Opinion about the best way to treat back pain is divided. Some recent studies show that fewer than 10 percent of people with severe back pain need surgery. The doctors who were sur-veyed believed that most injuries, strains, sprains, and even slipped discs will heal themselves in a matter of weeks.

The school of thought is that a few days of rest (no more than two or three days in bed), heat, physical therapy, swimming or walking, spinal manipulation, good nutrition, and over-the-counter pain relievers will relieve the pain, and regular exercise will keep the muscles and ligaments strong enough to prevent further back problems. These doctors do not recommend extensive, expensive tests such as magnetic resonance imaging, bone scans, CT scans, or myelograms, prescription pain relievers, steroids, or injections into the spine. Nor do they endorse acupuncture, traction, or Transcutaneous Electronic Nerve Stimulation.

That group of medical practitioners suggests that if severe pain continues unabated for more than three months, or if there is loss of bowel or bladder control, a sudden pronounced weakness of the legs, or tingling or numbness in them, surgery may be indicated and a thorough evaluation of the patient should be made.

The more traditional treatment for spinal injuries continues to be an early, thorough examination, including X rays at the very least. If further evaluation is indicated, the physicians may proceed with any or all of a full gamut of sophisticated, high-tech tests in order to define the problem accurately. They may prescribe muscle relaxants, prescription pain killers, traction, bed rest, or surgery.

More studies will undoubtedly be made, and considerable debate take place, before there is agreement on what is best for back injuries. Even then, there is probably not a single, specific treatment that is appropriate for everyone.

Chapter 23

COPING SOCIALLY

Strategies for coping with any of the problems of life are learned from watching how other people deal with them, or from being taught by someone, or through "burn-your-butt-and-sit-on-the-blister" experiences. It seems to take all of them for me to learn and I'm not sure I'll ever know all the ways of coping with pain. If there is anything you can take from the lessons I've learned and use it to help yourself, do it.

It surprised me to realize that, after being ill and attended to for as long as I was, my focus shifted from looking outward at the people around me to inward and too centered on myself. There were times when I hurt so badly that I couldn't think about anything else. Doctors and nurses paid attention to my every complaint. Friends rallied around me and surrounded me with affection and assistance. The man I loved held my hand and wiped away my tears. I was treated like a princess and I almost forgot that my prince and everyone else in the palace needed love and attention, too.

Now that I'm getting well, I'm attending to my friends better, phoning them and catching up on all of the news I missed, and seeing them socially. I'm listening to them more than I'm talking about myself and I'm letting them know how much they mean to me. I'm letting Stanford know, too, how much I treasure him and I want to make each one of his days a happy one.

My social activities are different from what they used to be and I'm trying to get used to that. Instead of participating in active outdoor sports with other people, I spend that time at the health club talking with friends while we work out, having them to my home for lunch or dinner, or going sight-seeing with them.

If there's a reception to attend I talk with the hostess in advance and explain that I'll need to sit down from time to time and I let her know that I'll probably have to leave early. That allows me to be in control of what I can physically manage and it makes the hostess happy that I cared enough to make the effort to come to her party.

When friends invite me to their house for the evening, it's with their blessing that I may get up from the chair, move around, and go home when I need to. When they come to my house, it's with the knowledge that it won't be a grand, elaborate, formal evening, just a happy, congenial, and comfortable time with good food for fine company. I think it must be all right: Bea said to me at the end of a birthday dinner I gave in her honor, "Let's not eat out anymore. Let's let you cook!"

An important aspect of my social life is breakfast with Stanford and I'm well enough now to prepare it at six o'clock every morning. Lunches and dinners are bonuses and so is hot popcorn and Saturday basketball on television. Bobby Knight is still coaching at Indiana University and it's fun to see those games.

My life is quite calm and sheltered compared to the way it used to be, and because of that my style of dressing is different. I'm no longer in the fashion industry or the social whirl so I don't have to wear every newest style or have perfectly coifed hair. Perfect hair and daily swimming don't go together very well anyway. I can be more relaxed about both my appearance and my behavior.

Do I miss my old way of life? Yes, a great deal. But I'm learning to like this one, too.

Chapter 24

COPING FINANCIALLY

Of all the coping I'm having to learn to do, finance is perhaps the most basic. All my life the greatest horror I could think of was for anyone to become old, ill, alone, and broke, all at the same time. I've done everything I've known to do to keep it from happening to me, and with the enormous losses caused by my back, I'll have to keep trying.

Financial advisors say a person should have enough liquid assets to take care of himself and his family for eight to twelve months without income. As difficult as it often was, I usually managed to divert a little money into a savings account on a regular basis. Yet it never crossed my mind that I'd ever be unable to work and would need to use my savings to support myself.

Now that I know about medical catastrophes and understand how it feels to watch my money disappear, thousands of dollars at a time, I believe more firmly than ever that most of us need to save money even when we think we can't afford to do it.

I also believe it's essential to be well insured, even if the costs of premiums pinch my budget. I didn't expect ever to file an insurance claim, and sometimes I thought I was managing my money poorly by owning medical policies, but then I learned that it was better for me always to be a little bit insurance poor than to be made destitute by a costly illness. You can imagine the financial condition I would be in at this time if it weren't for Blue Cross/Blue Shield, Workmen's Compensation

Insurance, and some small supplemental policies that I bought years and years ago when I was still insurable.

It might seem wasteful to you, but I find it's important for me to own bank cards, too, and to have the most generous credit limits they'll allow. The annual fees are minimal when compared with the security they provide me. Bank cards are my instant access to reserve funds in an emergency. There are no humbling trips to the loan officer at the bank, no loan applications to fill out, and no waiting for days while a committee reviews the application. With a bank card I have access to money without ever leaving the hospital or home. In most instances I pay off any charges within thirty days and that gives me access to the full credit amount all over again.

It's supremely important to me to conscientiously protect my credit rating. I scrutinize every bill I receive, especially medical bills, to make sure they're correct and haven't already been paid but not posted, and I write checks for my bills promptly. I want my credit history to be impeccable so that I have as much financial substance and power as I can. No one knows what the future may bring. During bad times people frequently say, "Oh, well. Things can't get any worse." It's not true. They *can*.

My nonspinal medical bills average about $350 a month, year after year, and insurance covers only a percentage of the cost. The medical costs directly related to my back have reached some $500,000, and I can't begin to calculate how much I've spent for mileage to medical appointments and for the paid services of people who have helped me at home. And I've probably lost a million dollars in future earnings because of the loss of my profession, and from closing Lucy's Pillowtalk.

Those facts make me try to be prudent with my money, particularly when I'm not yet able to work and don't now when, if ever, I will be able to work. I don't know how far my money will have to stretch. I don't want to be penurious, but neither do I want to go broke. I am coping financially, but I'm trying to learn to cope better and more easily.

Chapter 25

SURE, YOU CAN TRAVEL THOUGH HANDICAPPED!

It had been more than a year since I'd been to the ocean and I longed to smell the salt air, feel the ocean breeze on my face, and walk barefooted on the beach. When you're a Pisces living in the desert, you're gills dry out. Any seashore always has restorative powers for me and the pull of the sea becomes greater with each month that I'm away from it.

During relaxation exercises in the hospital I had mentally transported myself back to La Jolla in southern California. I'd sat in front of the huge, arched window at La Valencia Hotel and watched the palm trees and the Pacific Ocean, lunched on tropical fruit in the lush garden restaurant, stood on the cliffs along the shore as the swells smashed hard against the rocks, walked along the beach with sand in my toes, and explored the galleries and boutiques along the boulevard.

I talked with Stanford about a vacation I wanted to take. "It seems like a long time since I was at the ocean and I'd like to take a few days to go to La Jolla if I can figure out a way to travel comfortably. While I'm doing it I'd like to research the subject of traveling when you're handicapped and write a magazine article about it. It would be more fun if you came with me. Would you like to?" I asked. "Would you let me build you that day I promised? We could do anything and everything you want to."

"Yes, I'd like to, but I can't get away during the week. Why don't you go ahead and make the trip, write your article and get some sand in your toes, and I'll fly out for the weekend and come back with you?" he answered.

I phoned Frederick and Margaret Myers, who had been my friends and travel agents for a long time. We had also traveled together one summer when we took a group of sixty-four teenagers by ship to England and Europe. It's interesting that my first acquaintance with Dr. and Mrs. Schultz was at that time: their daughter went to Europe with us.

"Margaret, I really want to get away for a few days and get a new perspective on my life. I also want to research traveling as a handicapped person. If someone has several physical limitations, how difficult is it to travel by air? I'd like to book a flight to San Diego and lease a car to travel from there," I said into the phone.

"There's nothing to it. Thousands of people who are much older than you are and have disabilities far worse than yours travel every day. Tell me your limitations and we'll take care of everything. We'll book you with an airline that's known for meeting the individual needs of its passengers. What assistance do you think you'll need?" Margaret asked.

"First, I can't carry luggage, so I'll need to be sure of a skycap at the beginning and ending of the trip. I walk with a cane and I can't walk very far or stand in long lines. It bothers me to sit still for more than a half-hour, so I need a stopover to break the flight. Also I'm supposed to avoid the risk of hard bumps or falls."

"No problem," Margaret said. "Tell me what kind of car you want and where you want to stay. We'll go to work on it and call you back."

I didn't want to say it, but my biggest concern was my embarrassment at requesting special assistance both now and during the trip. Would I stand out too much? Would other passengers look at me in a wheelchair with sympathy or, even worse, disdain? I wanted so much just to be like everybody else! I needed a change of scene, but was the trip going to be an exhausting ordeal and not be worth what it would take?

I hadn't even finished worrying when Margaret phoned. "We

have you booked on an airline that will pay attention to your needs. A skycap will meet you at the curbside ticket counter, check your bags, and take you by wheelchair through the terminal to your departure gate. You're assigned an aisle seat in the first row behind the bulkhead so you'll have the most room to stretch and you won't have to climb over anyone to get out. You'll have a short layover in Phoenix where you can get off the plane and move around. When you land in San Diego, a skycap will meet you with a wheelchair and take you to the baggage-claim carousel, collect your bags, and take you to your car," she detailed.

That sounded like a trip I could manage.

"Your room at La Valencia overlooks the water and the reservation is guaranteed. Can you think of anything else you might need?" Margaret finished.

"No, it sounds great! Let's try it and see how it goes," I answered and thanked her.

On the day of departure Stanford dropped me at the streetside ticket counter and turned me over to the skycap. He greeted me brightly, tagged my bags, and brought a wheelchair. He cheerily wheeled me through quiet passageways away from the crowds and commotion in the terminal, which was undergoing a $120 million reconstruction and was a dusty, drafty, congested mess with construction workers carrying tools and building materials everywhere.

I asked the skycap to tell me about himself.

"Well," he began, "my name is Eddie Duarte. I have a degree in social work and I'm working on my master's in counseling at the University of New Mexico. And I love opportunities to help people."

"Do very many people with special needs travel?" I asked.

"Oh, yeah!" Eddie exclaimed. "All kinds. All ages. All the time."

"Do they ever seem self-conscious about the extra assistance they need?" I asked next.

"Yes, and it seems to be worse for the men. They can't wait to get out of this wheelchair and onto the plane!"

At the final check-in counter, Eddie turned me over to the agent, who confirmed my seat assignments for both segments of the flight and gave me a boarding pass. "I'll personally escort you to the plane during early boarding," he said generously, glancing at the wheelchair I had been sitting in.

"How far is it from here to the boarding gate?" I asked, speculating on whether I needed to get back into the wheelchair or if I could walk the rest of the way with the cane.

Jokingly the agent answered, "It's at Gate D. That's not all that bad. It could be worse, like Gate H." He began to walk with me, disregarding the wheelchair completely.

On board the plane the flight attendant stored my cane in an overhead compartment with everyone else's belongings and the plane took off. The flight to Phoenix was smooth, on schedule and short, and I felt great. Traveling by air is a piece of cake, I was thinking.

The layover in Phoenix was long enough for me to move around and limber up, stretch, and eat a light lunch. A new crew came on duty and confirmed, "A skycap will meet you with a wheelchair when we land in San Diego and he'll stay with you as long as you need him."

Sure enough, when we landed and the plane door opened, a skycap waited with two wheelchairs: one for me and one for a passenger who was breathing from an oxygen tank. There was no waiting as the skycap pushed us both simultaneously to the baggage-claim area, joking all the way.

"How was your flight?" he asked.

"Terrific! Smooth, fast, and really pleasant. I'm having a wonderful time!" I answered happily.

I was, too. There weren't any delays or hassles, no sympathetic glances from anyone, all of the attendants and agents were cheerful, and in all three terminals there were amputees on crutches, older people in wheelchairs, and people who carried their own oxygen supply, all traveling someplace. I didn't feel nearly as conspicuous as I thought I would. People were treating me just like anybody else.

At the baggage carousel the skycap disappeared for a long time. I was curious about the delay at first, but as the minutes rolled by I became concerned. What was he doing that was taking so long? I wondered. My car was waiting and I wanted to be on my way.

Looking frustrated and disgruntled, the skycap returned and said, "I'm sorry but your bags are lost. I talked with the baggage manager and he can't find them either. We don't know how it could have happened. The manager is coming to talk with you about it."

At that moment the manager walked over to us and introduced himself to me. "I don't know where your baggage is or how it got lost, but I've already phoned Phoenix and Albuquerque to trace it. Are you here for a vacation? Are you staying with friends?" he asked.

"Yes and no," I answered. "I'm staying at La Valencia Hotel in La Jolla and I'm here for pleasure, but I'm also doing the research to write an article for a travel magazine. The article is about how to take a safe, pleasant, problem-free plane trip even if you're handicapped."

"Oh my God!" the manager burst out and quickly glanced around to see if anyone was listening. "Look, don't use my name. I'll keep tracing your baggage and the moment it gets here I'll personally deliver it to you at your hotel! I'm more sorry for the inconvenience than I can tell you and I hope you have a good trip anyway."

I couldn't help but laugh at the situation. "My biggest wish was to be just like everybody else on this trip," I said to the two men, "but I didn't expect that lost luggage would be the common bond among us."

The manager and skycap grinned with relief that I wasn't irate. The manager shook my hand and left to trace the luggage and the skycap took me to the waiting car.

I did write the magazine article and summarized it with these suggestions for handicapped travelers:

TEN HINTS FOR HANDICAPPED TRAVELERS

1. Allow more time than usual before, between, and after flights so that skycaps can get their equipment and give you the assistance you need.

2. Airline personnel are notified in advance that you will need assistance. Remind them at each check-in and departure exactly what assistance you will need.

3. Tip appropriately for the skycap's increased time and work. He probably could earn numbers of other tips

during the time he gives to you alone.

4. If you take medications, divide them into two containers: put one in your luggage and carry one with you, including enough extra medication for two days longer than you think you'll be traveling.

5. Dress well. People look up to you more and offer their help more often.

6. Wear clothes that will work for several occasions in case your luggage is delayed.

7. Carry a snack if you are going to have a layover. There might not be food services close to the gate where you wait for your next flight.

8. Don't explain to attendants all the details of your physical problem unless it's critical for them to know. They will happily assist you without knowing everything about you.

9. Be cheerful and confident even if you feel uneasy. Other people will reflect back that cheerfulness and confidence and you'll feel better.

10. Expect to have a good time.

Chapter 26

IMAGE BECOMES REALITY

Not very many months ago, lying desperate in Intensive Care, I wanted only to die and end my misery. I didn't die. There were good reasons why I should live and resume a normal life, although I couldn't see them at the time.

Now much has changed: my health, my knowledge about how to take care of it, my determination to turn my dreams into reality, and my zest for life, as on this special day at a lush, green tropical terrace restaurant in La Jolla. I linger long over a lunch of fresh crab salad and juicy, exotic fruits. Then, rested and happy, I walk out to the beach and my winter-paled skin is touched with color from the brilliant sun.

Gratefully, I have no more need for the hospital split-back cotton gowns; instead I wear a brand-new swimsuit, emerald green and scandalously brief. The sky is clear and blue and a sea breeze blows and fluffs my hair as I stroll along the shore. I watch the lobstermen unload their traps from rusty trucks and stow them in old dinghies to begin their hunts.

Sun-warmed children build sand castles just above the line of lapping waves and kids in bright, brief swimsuits toss their beach balls up the shore. One by one the joggers, some young, others not, pass me with a greeting and a smile. A few yards out from the shore the scuba-diving students don their gear and, backwards, walk to deeper sea. Surfers, bobbing with the waves, wait for the biggest swells to rush in from Hawaii.

I watch the other lovers of the sea for just a little while, then walk across the beach, warm sand between my toes, and lay my cane beside a mossy rock beyond the high tide's reach. Little foamy waves send cold chills up my legs and splash me as they rush on up the sand.

I walk and swim into deep surf, my cane so far away. I'm glad. I bob with each new swell, watch far out to sea, and wait for one great wave to rumble toward me so that I can catch a ride up to the shore. I scan the sea and here it comes, a swell so huge it seems to grow to towering heights with rolls of white foam riding on its crest.

It's here! I raise my arms and face the shore, then leap to lay my body on the crest and capture one swift, sweet, ferocious ride. I laugh aloud and cry in happiness, salt tears mixed with salty sea.

I reach the shore and stretch my body on the warm, soft sand. Oh, God, thank you for that ride! It's so wonderful just to be me once more!

GOD, YOU WERE NEAR ME, WEREN'T YOU?

God, you were near me this whole time, weren't you? Are you going to reveal to me why it all happened and what I was supposed to learn from it? You wouldn't do this without some purpose, would you? You surely must have some grand design it all fits into that makes it worth what everyone went through. If there's something you want me to do, when are you going to let me know? And how? Sometimes I think you're hard to understand, but you'll find I am now listening again.

SEA-BORN PHILOSOPHY

There is a rhythm to the ocean,
A tempo of the soul,
A power to build a way of life
And reach a private goal.

In precious moments on the shore
I've learned a code for living;
Although the day be bright or black
I can continue giving.

I find it's true that I'm indebted
But no one owes to me.
I've no collections due from them;
Relationships are free.

Each tension, every problem,
That intrudes upon my life
Will hone my skills of coping
With the tragedies and strife.

And I must live all my todays
As though there's a tomorrow
Accountable for things I've done
With no regrets, no sorrow.

SUGGESTED READING

Not all problems are back problems. Here is some suggested reading for information and encouragement.

Barley, Betsy Gregg. "Stress and Disease." *Ladies' Home Journal,* May 1987.

Benton, Laura, Lucinda L. Baker, Bruce R. Bowman, and Robert L. Waters. *Functional Electrical Stimulation—A Practical Clinical Guide.* 2d ed. Downey, Calif.: Ranchos Los Amigos, 1981.

Berland, Theodore, and Robert G. Addison. *Living with Your Bad Back.* New York: St. Martin's Press, 1983.

Bradley, Denise J. *What Does It Feel Like to Have Diabetes: A Diary of Events in the Life of a Diabetic.* Springfield, Ill.: Charles C. Thomas, 1987.

Bradley-Steck, Tara. "Studies Find Optimism Is Stronger Than Expected." *Albuquerque Journal,* June 21, 1987.

Burns, David D., M.D. *Feeling Good: The New Mood Therapy.* New York: Avon Books, 1992.

Cailliet, Rene, M.D. *Understand Your Backache: A Guide to Prevention, Treatment, and Relief.* Philadelphia: F. A. Davis, Co., 1984.

Callahan, Steven. *Adrift: Seventy-six Days Lost at Sea.* New York: Ballantine Books, 1987.

Dachman, Ken, and John Lyons. *You Can Relieve Pain.* New York: HarperCollins, 1990.

Dickenson, Mollie. *Thumbs Up: The Jim Brady Story.* New York: William Morrow & Co., 1987.

Dougherty, Ronald J. "Transcutaneous Electrical Nerve

Stimulation: An Alternative to Drugs in the Treatment of Acute and Chronic Pain." Paper presented at the 34th Annual Scientific Assembly of the American Academy of Family Physicians, San Francisco, October 4-7, 1982.

Findlay, Steven. "Taking Control of Your Pain." *U.S. News and World Report* 112, June 15, 1992.

Future Youth: How to Reverse the Aging Process. Editor of Prevention Magazine Books. Emmaus, Pa.: Rodale Press, Inc., 1987.

Goald, Harold J. "Microlumbar Disectomy." *Virginia Medical Monthly,* August 1976.

Gordon, Barbara. *I'm Dancing As Fast As I Can.* New York: Bantam Books, 1980.

Heller, Joseph, and Speed Vogel. *No Laughing Matter.* New York: Avon Books, 1987.

Keim, Hugo A., M.D., and W. H. Kirkaldy-Willis, M.D. *Clinical Symposia: Low Back Pain.* Summit, N.J.: CIBA Pharmaceutical Company, 1980.

Kirkland, Gelsey. *Dancing On My Grave.* New York: Jove Publications, 1987.

Klein, Arthur C., and Dana Sobel. *Backache Relief.* New York: NAL/Dutton, 1986.

Klein, Elinor. "When Pain Is Your Partner." *Parade,* July 26, 1987.

Marcus, Norman J., and Jean S. Arbeiter. *Freedom from Chronic Pain.* New York: Simon & Schuster, 1994.

Matthews-Simonton, Stephanie, O. Carl Simonton, and James L. Creighton. *Getting Well Again.* New York: Bantam Books, 1978.

Peterson, Norma. "Mind Over Disease: II. Warning! Daily Hassles Are Hazardous!" *Reader's Digest,* April 1987.

Roark, Anne. "Pain: You Don't Have to Suffer." *McCall's* 119, July 1992.

Robinson, Donald. "Mind Over Disease: I. Your Attitude Can Make You Well." *Reader's Digest,* April 1987.

Root, Leon, M.D. *No More Aching Back: Dr. Root's New 15-Minute-*

a-Day Program for a Healthy Back. New York: Random House, 1990.

Sarno, John. *Mind Over Back Pain*. New York: Berkley Publishing, 1987.

Schatzil, Pullig. "Gentle Relief from the Back Stabbers." *Prevention* 45, February 1993.

Shaevitz, Marjorie Hansen. *The Superwoman Syndrome*. New York: Warner Books, 1988.

Shipko, Stuart. "Stress Itself Can Be Addictive." *Albuquerque Journal*, July 4, 1987. Copyright *Shape* magazine.

Sjolund, Bengt H., and Margareta B. Eriksson. *Endorphins and Analgesia Produced by Peripheral Conditioning Stimulation*. New York: Raven Press, 1979.

Spiegel, David. *Living Beyond Limits: A Scientific Mind-Body Approach to Facing Life-Threatening Illness*. New York: Random House, 1993.

Sternbach, Richard A., M.D. *Mastering Pain: A Twelve-Step Program for Coping with Chronic Pain*. New York: Ballantine Books, 1988.

Swertlow, Mary Murphy. "Conquering Her World of Pain." *Los Angeles Times Magazine*, October 4, 1987.

Switzer, E. E. "You Don't Have to Live With Pain." *New Choices for Retirement Living* 32, April 1992.

Taylor, Elizabeth. *Elizabeth Takes Off: On Weight Gain, Weight Loss, Self-Image, and Self-Esteem*. New York: G. P. Putnam's Sons, 1987.

Tollison, C. David. *Managing Chronic Pain: A Patient's Guide*. New York: Sterling Publishing Co., Inc., 1979.

University of California, Berkeley. *Wellness Letter* 4, no. 6 (March 1988).

SUGGESTED LISTENING
FOR RELAXATION

Accelerating Self-Healing.

Breathe. Jon Bernoff and Marcus Allen. The Art of Relaxation. Vital Body Marketing Co., Inc., Box 1067, Manhasset, N.Y. 11030, 1985.

Carmel by the Sea. Pacific Ocean Surf. Electrifying Thunderstorms. A Sun Filled Stream. The Musical Sea of Tranquility. The Cry of the Loon. Sounds and Songs of the Humpback Whale. Sounds of a Crackling Fireplace. Sounds of the Tropical Rain Forest. The Romantic Sea of Tranquility. Sounds of Nature Sampler. Pachelbel Canon with Sounds of the Ocean Surf. Gentle Persuasion/The Sounds of Nature. The Special Music Company, 87 Essex St., Hackensack, N.J. 07801, 1991.

Collage. Psycho-Acoustical Laboratories, Inc., 10-45 Forty-eighth Ave., Long Island City, N.Y. 11101.

Country Stream. Desert Moon Sounds. Enhancing . . .

Environments: New Concepts in Stereo Sound, Cassette 1. Atlanta Recording Corp., 75 Rockefeller Plaza, N.Y. 10019.

Forest and the Water, The.

Gentle Rain.

Getting Well. Carl Simonton, M.D., D.A.B.R. Audio Renaissance Tapes, Inc., 9110 Sunset Blvd., Ste. 240, Los Angeles, Calif. 90069.

Musical Sleep Induction. Dr. Robert Sohn and Jim Oliver. Mindbody, Inc. Third Ear Music, distributed by Vital Body

Marketing Co., Inc., Box 1067, Manhasset, N.Y. 11030.

Mystic Sea, The.

Ocean Surf.

Pain Management. Health Talk Self-health Tapes and Informa-
tion Booklet. UCLA Ext. Dept. of Health Sciences and UCLA
School of Medicine. Health Talk, P. O. Box 114-H, Grand
Haven, Mich. 49417.

Pastels. Georgia Kelly. The Art of Relaxation. Vital Body Marketing Co., Inc., Box 1067, Manhasset, N.Y. 11030, 1985.

Piano Meditation. Jim Oliver. The Art of Relaxation. Vital Body
Marketing Co., Inc., Box 1067, Manhasset, N.Y. 11030, 1985.

Relax: Subliminally Yours. Steven Halpern. The Art of Relaxation.
Vital Body Marketing Co., Inc., Box 1067, Manhasset, N.Y.
11030, 1985.

Relaxation by the Sea. Dr. Robert Sohn. The Art of Relaxation.
Vital Body Marketing Co., Inc., Box 1067, Manhasset, N.Y.
11030, 1985.

Rosewood and Silver. Vance Koenig and Warren Weisbach. The
Art of Relaxation. Vital Body Marketing Co., Inc., Box 1067,
Manhasset, N.Y. 11030, 1985.

Sailing: Nature's Answer to Stress. Ambient Psychoacoustics. The
Art of Relaxation. Vital Body Marketing Co., Inc., Box 1067,
Manhasset, N.Y. 11030, 1985.

Sea, The. Ambient Psychoacoustics. The Art of Relaxation.
Actual Sounds of Nature. Vital Body Marketing Co., Inc., Box
1067, Manhasset, N.Y. 11030, 1985.

Simple Gifts. Slow Ocean. Soothing Solo Piano.

Sound Health. Steven Halpern. The Art of Relaxation. Vital Body
Marketing Co., Inc., Box 1067, Manhasset, N.Y. 11030, 1985.

Sound Sleep. Steven Halpern. Musical Massage, A Soothing Sen-
sual Collection, Vol. 1. The Art of Relaxation. Vital Body Marketing Co., Inc., Box 1067, Manhasset, N.Y. 11030, 1985.

Stress Reduction. Health Talk Self-health Tapes and Information
Booklet. UCLA Ext. Dept. of Health Sciences and UCLA

School of Medicine. Health Talk, P.O. Box 114-H, Grand Haven, Mich. 49417.

Subliminal Relief of Back Pain. Subliminal Persuasion Self-hypnosis Cassette Tape. Potentials Unlimited, Inc., 4808-H Broadmoor SE, Grand Rapids, Mich. 49508, 1978.

Tempestuous Sea, The.

Timeless Sea, The.

You Are the Ocean. Schawkie Roth. The Art of Relaxation. Vital Body Marketing Co., Inc., Box 1067, Manhasset, N.Y. 11030, 1985.

SUGGESTED VIDEOS FOR RELAXATION

Back Pain. Dr. J. Knirk. American Medical Information, Video Consultation Series.

Feeling Good with Arthritis. Dr. Alan Kenakis. Kenajenex Productions, Andover, Mass. 01810.

No More Back Pain. Dr. Robert L. Swezey. Cequal Products, Inc., c/o The Swezey Institute, 1328 Sixteenth St., Santa Monica, Calif. 90404.

Relaxation. Barrie Konicov. Potentials Unlimited Subliminal Persuasion Video, Grand Rapids, Mich.

Walk Without Pain. Florida Spine Institute, 2250 Drew St., Clearwater, Fla. 34625.

Water Colors. Pete Bardens. BMG Music Video, 1133 Avenue of the Americas, New York, N.Y. 10036.

INDEX

Acupressure, 200
Acupuncture, 32, 200
Addison's disease, 65
Adhesive tape, 100
Administration, 61, 66, 68, 69, 195
Adrenal insufficiency, 100
Advanced Neurological Unit, 106, 107, 109, 135
AIDS, 60, 118, 119
Albuquerque, 22, 38, 76, 79, 125, 126, 162, 168, 189, 215
Albuquerque Country Club, 162
Allergies, 36, 100, 106, 108, 120
Allopurinol®, 100
All-or-nothing syndrome, 163, 176
Anesthesiologist, 91, 105, 106, 130, 135
Anesthetic, 42, 47, 91, 105, 106, 108, 130, 181
Anna Kaseman Hospital, 82, 95
Antibiotics, 100
Anti-inflammatories, 100
Appendectomy, 100
Atlantic Recording Corporation, 200

Bank cards, 210
Barrow, Wess, 33, 37, 107, 118, 125, 132-35, 143, 148-49

Beck Inventory, 113
Benadryl®, 88, 124, 132, 142
Biofeedback, 178, 179
Bittner, Barnett, 33, 37-39, 49, 78, 107, 115, 119, 120, 135, 149, 150
Bittner, Beatrice, 33, 37-39, 49, 68, 78, 81, 82, 107, 115, 116, 119, 120, 135, 149, 150, 208
Bittner, Ruth, 120
Blood, 22-24, 58, 95, 96, 117-19, 126, 133, 137, 138, 142, 178
Blood donations, 118
Blood sugar, 95, 96
Blood transfusions, 117, 118
Blood type, 117, 118
Bone scan, 23-25, 84, 87, 88, 205
Bowels, 23, 139
Brack Center, 76
Brain scan, 82
Brodie, Jim, 93
Bull Ring Restaurant, 170
Burns, David, 40, 115
Buscaglia, Leo, 36, 196

California Gift Show, 76
Chicago, 40, 77, 120
Child abuse, 31, 69, 81
Children of a Lesser God, 162
Chiropractor, 32
Coley, Art, 93

Cook County Hospital, 40
Coping, 73, 112, 116, 183, 186, 204, 210, 219; emotionally, 193; financially, 209; physically, 199; socially, 207
Copp, Steven N., 17
Cortisone, 100, 130, 154, 182, 204; Acetate®, 100; ointment, 182; solution, 106, 130, 141
Counseling, 21, 42, 57, 66, 69, 127, 213
CT scan, 23, 42, 84, 87, 88, 187, 205

Dallas Trade Mart, 78
Daskalos, Pete, 97
Dear Abby, 189-91
Depo-Estradiol®, 100
Designer Showcase, 93
Dillon, Rev. Austin, 33, 37, 98
Disc, 25, 27, 28, 43, 51, 52, 138; ruptured, 51-52
Discussion groups, 69, 183
Diuretics, 154-55
Dixon, George, 94
Dobkins, D. A., 193
Dobkins, Terry, 134, 138
Duarte, Eddie, 213

Ecotrin®, 100
Electrical stimulation machine, 58
Employee benefits, 74
Endocrine system, 44, 65
Endocrinologist, 74, 79, 82, 96, 106, 204
Endorphins, 202
England, 40, 63, 212
Epidural blocks, 90. See also Nerve blocks
Estrogen, 74, 204
Exercises, isometric, 159, 199

Faith healers, 98
Fallopian tubes, 100
Fame Time, 93
Farnum, Myrna, 93
Fearn, Leif, 68
Feeling Good, 115
Fiber-optic cable, 97, 98
First United Methodist Church, 37, 65, 98
Foot brace, 74
Foot drop, 50, 56, 94, 186
Foster, Dee, 39, 56, 98, 127, 128, 135
Fouch, Forrest, 60, 84

Genetics, 67, 196
Gerardo, Harriet, 87
Gifted children, classes for, 35, 66, 68, 69
Glasser, William, 69
Golden State Warriors, 52
Goodsell, Marilyn, 93, 134
Gout, 100, 186
Grady, Gilbert, 35, 89, 131, 136, 138, 142, 144
Griego, Genara, 182, 183
Grivas, Peter, 77, 125, 196

Hall, Stanford, 21, 33, 36, 38, 39, 44-47, 49, 50, 53-57, 62-64, 67, 69, 70, 73, 75-80, 82, 83, 87, 89-93, 102, 107, 118-20, 126, 133-36, 139, 141, 143, 144, 148-51, 153, 154, 164, 168-73, 175, 176, 180, 183, 189, 196, 197, 200, 207, 208, 211, 213
Handicapped people, 157, 158, 163, 168, 203, 211-16; handicap license plate, 158, 168, 203; handicap parking, 157, 168; handicapped travelers, 211-16

Hanratty, Virginia, 99-101, 135, 145

Harrison, Rosemary, 89

Heat, 32, 51, 114, 205

Heights General Hospital, 68

Herpes zoster, 182. *See also* Shingles)

Hester, Reid, 112-16, 124, 126-28, 143, 147, 148, 159-63, 167, 177-79, 203

Hiatus hernia, 100

Hilgers, Josi, 21-23

"Hispanic Christmas" (poem), 200

Hoffman, Dolores, 126

Hoffman, James, 126

Hollinger, Gail, 163

Home Health Care, 39, 45

Hong Kong, 195. *See also* Raichandani, Lachmi

Hormones, 204

Hot spots, 24, 88

Hot tub, 203

Hurley, Lloyd, 35, 48, 89, 131, 164

Hypoglycemia, 96

Hypogonadism, 100

Hypopituitarism, 100

Hypothyroidism, 65, 100

Ice treatments, 32, 142, 173

Indiana University, 50-52, 208

"I Need a New Life, God," 64

Insulin, 92, 96, 118

Insurance, 32, 49, 74, 99, 159, 168-70, 209, 210

Intensive Care, 92, 106-8, 135, 136, 139, 141, 217

Jo, Rashi, 91

Kaplan, Ralph, 94, 95, 101, 109, 111, 112, 117, 121, 124, 129

Kassam, Shiraz, 97

Katz, Simon, 93

Khalsa, Sarb Sarang Kaur, 153, 158, 175, 180, 202

Kitchel, Barbara, 53

Kitchel, Edwin, 50, 51, 96

Kitchel, Ted, 50-54, 61, 143

Knight, Bobby, 50, 208

Kuala Lumpur, Malaysia, 67

La Cienega, 171, 175

La Jolla, California, 211, 215, 217

Lash, Sally, 102

La Valencia Hotel (La Jolla), 211, 215

Levothroid®, 100

Life Line program, 68

Link, The, 38

Loew's Anatole Hotel (Dallas), 78

Los Angeles Clippers, 52

Los Angeles Mart, 76

Lucy's Pillowtalk, 77, 83, 101, 204, 210

Lung, collapsed, 138

Magdich, Dennis, 77

Magnesium gluconate, 100

Magnetic Resonance Imaging, 186, 205. *See also* MRI exam

Managing Chronic Pain: A Patient's Guide, 115

Manganese, 100

Manzano del Sol retirement center, 133-34

March, Edris, 93

Massage, 58, 200

Maxide®, 100

Maydew, Randy, 105, 106

Medical costs, 198, 210

Medications, 44, 47, 74, 79, 100, 106, 107, 109, 114, 124, 141, 144, 147, 182, 183, 204, 216
Medoff, Mark, 162
Menswear Mart, 78
Michaels, June, 98
Microsurgery, 51
Millon Behavior Health Inventory, 113
Milwaukee Bucks, 53
Mind Over Back Pain, 162
"Mind Over Disease," 202
Minerals, 74, 100, 142, 204
Minnesota Multiphasic Personality Inventory (MMPI), 113, 114
Mitchell, William, 106, 144, 181-83
Moloney, Agnes, 40
Mora, Federico, 46-48, 84, 87-89, 92, 94, 181, 186-88
Moslem Mosque, 97
Motor Vehicle Department, 203
MRI exam, 186-88, 193
Muscle relaxants, 32, 51, 205
Myelogram, 52, 87, 130, 132
Myers, Frederick, 98, 212
Myers, Margaret, 212, 213

National Basketball Association, 53
Nerve blocks, 90, 91
Nerve root decompressions, 47, 48, 84, 95, 99, 100, 103, 105, 107, 117, 129
Nerves, 23, 25, 27, 28, 32, 45, 50-52, 56-58, 84, 89-91, 109, 111, 124, 145, 181-82, 186-87; regeneration of, 74
Neurological examination, 181
Neurological Unit, 99, 106, 107, 109, 135

Neuroma, on ear, 154
Neurosurgeon, 46, 51, 52, 84, 89, 94, 96, 108
New Mexico Personnel and Guidance Association, 68
New Mexico State Department of Education, 66
New Mexico state insurance commissioner, 168, 169
New Mexico state legislature, 69, 128
Niame, 58
Northwestern University Hospital, 120
Nutrition, 142, 200, 205
Nystatin®, 100

Optimism, 49
Orthofuse, 29, 42, 43, 59, 100
Orthopedic Unit, 38, 49
Osteoarthritis, degenerative, 100
Osteoporosis, 74

Pain, 21-23, 32, 36, 45, 51-53, 59, 73, 78, 81, 83, 88, 94, 98, 99, 107-9, 112-15, 120, 121, 123, 124, 132, 133, 136-38, 142, 143, 149, 151, 153, 154, 158, 162, 165, 176-79, 181, 185, 186, 190, 193, 194, 197, 199, 200, 202-5, 207; control of pain, 114, 162; cocktails, 124; relief, 108, 139, 151, 181, 203-4
Palace of the Governors (Santa Fe), 169
Papaya extract, 32
Paramedics, 22, 23
Phoenix, 213-15
Physical therapists, 36, 37, 39, 110, 119, 121, 128, 144, 147, 199, 200

Physical therapy, 32, 58, 114, 121, 143, 177, 186, 205
Potassium, 100, 130, 154
Prayers, 97, 98
Pre-op, 106, 135
Progesterone, 204

Radiologist, 23, 25, 32, 88, 130
Radiology Unit, 88, 130, 132
Raichandani, Lachmi, 195, 196
Reader's Digest, 202
Relaxation, 36, 115, 121, 122, 179, 196, 200, 211
Respiratory Unit, 138
Restrictions, 41, 76
Retirement, 70, 74, 75, 80, 93, 134
Robert O. Anderson School of Business (University of New Mexico), 80
Rosett, Randy, 135

St. Aidan's Episcopalian Church, 98
St. George Greek Orthodox Church, 97
St. Joseph Hospital, 22, 49, 59, 84, 87, 90, 98, 129
Sanchez, Sandy (hairdresser), 133
Sandia National Labs, 126
San Diego, 69, 212-14
San Diego State University, 69
Santa Fe, 75, 121, 125, 167-72, 175, 196, 203
Sarno, John, 162
Sauna, 203
Scher, Jeanne, 35, 196
Schneider, Dirk and Jan, 180
Schultz, Sidney, 23-25, 31, 32, 35, 36, 38, 39, 41-43, 46, 47, 57-61, 63, 69, 70, 73, 74, 83, 84,

87-89, 92, 94, 95, 129-32, 136, 143-45, 148, 149, 154, 164, 165, 167, 176, 181, 185-88, 203, 212
Sciatic nerve, 51, 52
"Sea-Born Philosophy," 218
Seashore, 200, 211
Sex, 149, 204
Shaevitz, Marjorie Hansen, 160
Shingles, 182, 186
Should-ought syndrome, 161
Sick leave, 32, 59
Silent partner, 76, 77, 79, 80, 87, 89-90, 92, 195
Spinal fluid, 24, 25, 88
Spinal fusion, 25, 31-33, 35, 38, 42, 43, 47, 51, 52, 84, 88, 89, 92, 95, 100, 109, 114, 117, 129-31, 143, 145, 164, 165, 177, 179, 195; anterior, 89, 95, 129, 130, 143, 164, 165; cervical, 32, 100; non-union, 84, 88
Spinal stenosis, 28, 29, 84, 88, 89, 92, 95
Spironolactone®, 100
Steam room, 203
Stress, tension, 32, 36, 44, 113, 115, 121, 122, 133, 149, 152, 162, 165, 177-79, 196, 200, 202-4, 219
Stress fractures, 32
Sulfinpyrazone®, 100
Superwoman syndrome, 115, 157, 159, 160, 194
Swimming, 32, 59, 74, 126, 164, 165, 167, 186, 200, 205, 208
Swinson, Jo Ann, 58
Sympathetic dystrophy, 90, 100

Tafoya, Henry, 97, 125
Tanoan Country Club, 163
Tavist-1®, 100

Ten hints for handicapped travelers, 215-16
TENS Unit, 120, 121, 188
Testosterone, 204
Threet, Martin E., 44
Toes, 57, 58, 73, 90, 145; broken, 32
Tollison, C. David, 115
Tonsillectomy, 100
Traction, 32, 205
Transcutaneous Electronic Nerve Stimulation. See TENS Unit
Traveling when handicapped, 211-16
Trieste, Italy, 53
Tulane School of Social Work, 38

UCLA, 69
Ultrasound, 51, 181
Unitarian church, 98
United Blood Services, 117
University of New Mexico, 80, 195, 213
University of Pittsburgh, 197
Uric acid, 186

Vaginal bleeding, 182
Van Buren, Abigail. See Dear Abby
Vertebrae, 23-27, 29, 32, 43, 48, 51, 60, 73, 84, 91, 100, 131, 136, 137; fused, 73, 136;
lumbar, 25, 27, 32, 100; sacro, 100
Vertigo, 154, 155
Vital signs, 22, 39, 91, 103, 106, 130, 134
Vitamins, 74, 100, 142, 204

Waterbed, 153, 202, 203
Weight, 36, 74, 82, 91, 100, 119, 137, 142, 143, 153, 158, 164, 200
Williams, Darlene, 101, 112, 123, 124, 126, 149
Wingfield, Tom, 80, 81, 90, 93, 98, 133, 196
"Winter Clam Beds," 200, 201-2
Women's Apparel Mart, 78
Word processor, 180
World Bank of Good Deeds, 40
World Trade Center, 78
Wyndham Hotel (Dallas), 79

X rays, 23-25, 42, 60, 73, 82, 84, 87, 88, 130, 132, 137, 165, 177, 186, 187; chest, 23, 82; spinal, 23; technician, 23, 60, 132

Zantac®, 100
Zander, Emily, 195
Zartman, David, 65, 93, 115
Zartman, James K., 65, 93, 196
Zartman, Mary K., 63, 93, 134